10-Step Pilates

10-Step

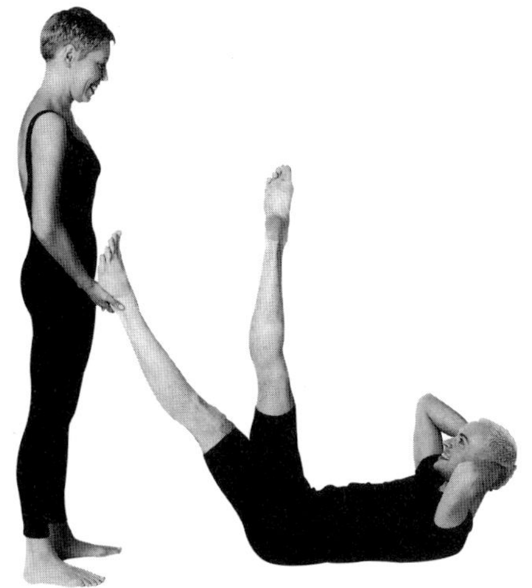

Pilates

Lesley Ackland with
Thomas Paton and
Malu Halasa

Thorsons
An Imprint of HarperCollins*Publishers*
77–85 Fulham Palace Road,
Hammersmith, London W6 8JB

The Thorsons website address is:
www.thorsons.com

Published by Thorsons 1999

10 9 8 7 6 5 4 3 2

Lesley Ackland and Thomas Paton assert the moral right to be identified as the authors of this work

A catalogue record for this book is available from the British Library

ISBN 0 7225 3936 3

Designed by Roger Hammond

Printed and bound in Great Britain by
Woolnough Bookbinding Ltd,
Irthlingborough, Northamptonshire

By Lesley Ackland:
15-Minute Pilates

In 1988 Lesley Ackland founded the Pilates-based Body Maintenance Studio at Pineapple Dance Studios, in London's Covent Garden. She was the Remedial Exercise Consultant to the Birmingham Royal Ballet for five years. Her first book, *15-Minute Pilates*, was published in 1998. *10-Step Pilates* is her second book for Thorsons.

Thomas Paton, former Royal Ballet dancer, currently performs in West End productions.

My best thanks to the talented writer, Malu Halasa, who helped make this book what it is.

Also a big thank you to Islay Sullivan, Chartered Physiotherapist and former Head of Physiotherapy to Birmingham Royal Ballet who was consultant on my first book and whose help is greatly appreciated.

If you have any enquiries regarding Body Maintenance Studios, please send a large SAE to:

Body Maintenance,
2nd Floor Pineapple,
7 Langley Street,
Covent Garden,
London WC2H 9JA

This book is dedicated to my mother, who has achieved the impossible and never been defeated by life.

Contents

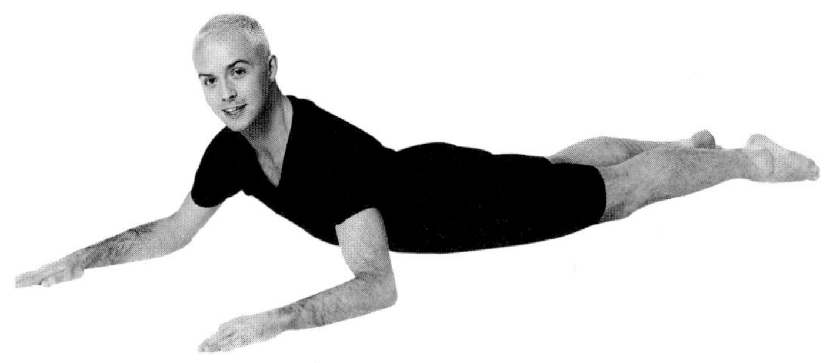

Introduction

Body awareness

With this Pilates-based Body Maintenance programme you can transform your body throughout the day, every day. *10-Step Pilates* describes straightforward exercises based on posture, breathing and visualization that will give you a longer, leaner figure, and a strong, well-toned body.

Designed to be practised at home, during a lunch break or before a big night out, the exercise programme in *10-Step Pilates* addresses fundamental questions about standing, sitting, moving and breathing. It promises no quick fixes or sudden improvements. However, with concentration and commitment, the end result will be rewarding and nothing short of enhanced physical and mental well-being.

Many people do not have a positive body self-image. Women, specifically, have a tendency to retreat from their bodies as they get older.

10-Step Pilates can help you achieve the body that you want – and are comfortable with, not the body someone else has judged to be more acceptable. Too often we are held hostage to figures in glossy magazines, imagining them to be preferable and easily attainable. I find this unrealistic, even dangerous. We should acknowledge and appreciate our own bodies and work with what we are naturally given. Many people do not even consider the highly desirable aspects of themselves. In this 'media-friendly' generation we are almost brainwashed into acknowledging 'the perfect body' hype, which is, in fact, merely the fashion of the moment. This can result in feelings of dissatisfaction and depression. We have the ability to transform ourselves, to reduce our self-imposed limitations and tap into our potential – using my techniques on a daily basis will stretch both the mind and the body.

Very few of us are born with an anatomically perfect body. Through habitual misuse, which begins when we are quite young and continues until we feel discomfort, we can seriously damage parts of the body. Unknowingly, certain areas are accentuated and, as we get older, it is more than likely that one side of the spine will be visibly over-developed. This is when problems manifest themselves. My *10-Step Pilates* attempts to create the best body on the frame that is possible for you, with the understanding that there is no such thing as the perfect body. All of us have imbalances. The trouble begins when an imbalance turns into a physical problem.

The Origins of Pilates

Although Pilates has been a technique traditionally used by injured dancers, it was a well-kept secret in old Hollywood, among the likes of Katharine Hepburn and Lauren Bacall. In the last few years there has been a rise in the number of Pilates studios from Hollywood to New York, and younger celebrities from Madonna to Uma Thurman and Courteney Cox have become avowed Pilates devotees. In a business where so much emphasis is placed on youthful-looking bodies, Pilates' leaner, longer look is very much in vogue.

Pilates was originally developed by Josef Pilates, a sickly child who began body-building at 14 to ward off tuberculosis. Later he incorporated a system of gentle physical exercise, which further strengthened his muscles, realigned his body and allowed him to overcome his problems to become a gymnast, boxer and circus performer. His exercises were developed in the 1920s, and they addressed the physical problems of his age. He first used pulleys and springs attached to hospital beds to stop muscle wastage among bedridden, injured troops during the First World War. Interned in Britain, he maintained that his exercise regime protected him and others from the dreaded Spanish Flu epidemic. Afterwards, in Germany, the dancer and choreographer Rudolph von Laban incorporated Pilates techniques of limbering and warm-up into his own dance method.

In the US, Pilates opened a studio in New York City, and it wasn't long before Balanchine brought injured dancers from the New York City Ballet to him for therapy. Using the Pilates technique, they were able to work through their injuries and increase their stamina while strengthening their bodies. Pilates has helped former Royal Ballet dancers like Thomas Paton, my co-author, and Nick Ringham, an associate and instructor at my Body Maintenance Studio. Thomas, who currently performs in West End productions, writes about his own experiences in the chapter entitled 'A Dancer's Life'. Nick, who began his Pilates training in 1987, reviews the method's key concepts in the chapter called 'Pilates Master Class'.

Pilates and Dancers

Pilates is for everyone, but it has become an important exercise regime for people who rely on their bodies for their careers. Although I've taught modern dancers, even athletes, historically Pilates has been linked with classical dance because of the relationship between Josef Pilates and Balanchine. As a remedial technique for classical dancers at the highest level, it is also used by top ballet companies. If there is even a hint of a physical problem, dancers go and do Pilates.

When injured, athletes and dancers can't afford to stop exercising altogether because muscle wastage would develop in the rest of their bodies and it would take them even longer to get back into shape. With Pilates you can exercise your body even if your leg is in a splint or in a cast. If you have a back problem and you're wearing a corset you can carry on doing Pilates to avoid muscle wastage in your legs. The method has been essential for classical dancers, who have used this method since its creation.

A major difference between people who rely on their bodies for their careers and people who don't is that dancers and athletes usually have a physiotherapist on hand, either in their companies or on their teams, or have access to constant medical attention. They also have a confidence in their bodies that most people just don't have. For many of us it can be quite frightening to adjust our minds to the fact that we can carry on exercising even when we're seriously injured or in constant pain. It's a mind set. Dancers and athletes have it mainly due to the medical back-up the rest of the population simply hasn't got. Some dancers may have physiotherapy every day.

Body Maintenance

Sixty years after Pilates was created, physical ailments have changed, but pain has not. Contemporary stress has induced a variety of debilitating afflictions. In 1980 I began developing Body Maintenance, a balanced system of exercise, body shaping and tone combined with mental improvement and nutrition, based on Pilates. I initially studied with Alan Herdman, who first brought Pilates to the UK. Then I began travelling regularly to New York City to study Pilates there. During my instruction abroad I became aware of a new wave of research on the human body, and I found myself looking at the way physiotherapists were working, particularly at the New York City Ballet with physio balls and Dynabands. I had also become aware of other forms of bodywork, including Feldenkreis and the Alexander Technique.

With Pilates as the main base, I began to integrate methods from a wide variety of sources, including remedial massage, osteopathy and injury clinics, and created my own unique system of bodywork, which I call Body Maintenance. During the last 11 years in my own studio at Pineapple Dance Studios in London's Covent Garden, I have worked successfully with people who have suffered from a variety of modern infirmities: RSI (carpel tunnel syndrome), chronic back pain (some of which stems from spinal surgery), HIV-related problems, aerobic sprains, extreme obesity, even low self-esteem.

Often called 'yoga with machines', the Pilates-based exercises in my studio often incorporate balls, ropes, springs and pulleys. However, the most important and long-lasting work takes place on the floor. Mat exercises, essential to body mobility and endurance, target weak, under-utilized muscles in the abdomen, lower back, arms and legs. Based on mat work, I devised the exercises for *10-Step Pilates* – straightforward, concentrated movements that don't require a gym or special equipment. What they do require are a few minutes: in the morning, during lunch and later in the evening. This is a complete exercise regime devised for individuals who might not have the inclination or opportunity to seek out my studio, but who want to benefit from my tried and proven Pilates-based Body Maintenance programme.

A Strong Centre

Today people are more preoccupied by their mental and psychological states than they are with the condition of their bodies. Because this split between mind and body has never been more pronounced, depression and obsessions, including eating disorders, have become commonplace. Subsequently, the only way for some people to connect with the physical aspect in their lives is through high-impact aerobics, running on a treadmill for hours or starving themselves. Shock methods are never successful. It is only under the conditions of gradual development, concentration and dedication that the body can be influenced in the long term.

In many Eastern religions, the centre of the body is not the heart, but the pelvis. In Pilates, all things are possible from a strong core of the body, which is the stomach or abdominal muscles. By centring, concentrating and coordinating, *10-Step Pilates* will give your body a new awareness. Every time you stand up and walk you are carrying that different body. Each time you move, your limbs react in a new way. This is linked to the different way in which your pelvis sits on top of your legs, and the way in which your shoulder girdle is realigned. More than a physical activity, *10-Step Pilates* is a lifestyle change.

Many of us spend our time sitting at a desk, staring at a computer screen. As a result physical mobility has been lost. These exercises are designed to allow your body to return to its natural shape, particularly in the way the joints are realigned.

Liberation through Exercise

There can be a liberation and a spontaneity through exercise, but this initial release can only be achieved through practice and careful reprogramming of your body, which gets rid of 'negative baggage'. By this I mean anything from falling out of a tree when you were three – it can be something as simple as that – to being bullied at school because you were too tall, or breaking an ankle when you were skiing, or even having major spinal surgery at 25.

When I exercise I am balancing and harmonizing all the areas in my body so I can create the lightness and spontaneity of a child. By releasing tension through the correct use of exercise, you balance and integrate your body in the way you walk, the lightness in your step and the freedom in your muscles and joints.

Looking and Feeling Good

In every physical activity there is always a mental complement. Integrated into a daily routine, *10-Step Pilates* has another dimension that goes beyond the muscle toning and lengthening. The resulting physical lightness will engender a mental lightness as well, and this juncture is crucial. Feeling good about yourself and how you look enables your body and mind to meet harder challenges and make more gains. Positive thoughts inevitably bring about positive change.

People often come to me and say they hate their stomachs, over-developed thighs or flabby arms. From my experience, a poor self-image usually manifests itself physically somewhere in the body. Observing the way people walk, how they talk and interact with others, I can tell if they are closed, tense, isolated.

Virtually everyone has similar problems. It is easy for me to look at people's bodies and see that they have tight gluteals – the muscle group around the buttocks – tight hamstrings, or a weak, tight lower back, weak abdominals or tight hip flexors. Many people have rounded shoulders. They don't use their shoulder blades and *Latissimus Dorsi*, the muscles beneath the shoulder blades. They don't understand that the *Scapulae*, the shoulder blades, should glide. They do everything from Clavicle Elevation – the lifting of the shoulders – to the rounding of their shoulders, and end up with a forward pointing head, uncomfortable tight neck muscles, and the entire body completely out of alignment. To fight this feeling of falling forward all the time they contract their buttocks, which basically sends negative energy down through the back of the legs. The pelvis and feet are tight as well. You have as many bones in your feet as you have in the rest of your body, and yet people routinely neglect to exercise their feet.

The release of energy that takes place during *10-Step Pilates* dissipates stress, tightness and internalized aggression. The more you start to think about your breath, your energy and yourself as a complete, integral human spirit, the more you will be able to think of the way you present yourself to others and the way you accept yourself. By integrating the sense of body, mind and spirit together, you create the person you wish to be together with what you want to achieve on a physical level.

The Stress of Ageing

Age and gravity are constantly dragging us down. For men and women, the notion of ageing is deeply ingrained not only in our consciousness but in popular culture. It may be difficult to think about ageing in a positive way, but some people are comfortable within themselves. They've said to me, 'I am going to be true to myself and who I want to be today, and not be cast in how I looked 10 years ago.' Or 'When I become middle-aged, I don't have to mirror the way my parents were at the same age.'

With new research in physiology and anatomy, fear of ageing is counter-productive. We know how the body works. Essentially what you put in – whether it's physical activity, diet or nutrition – is what you get out. If you are physically heavy and out of touch, your body feels tired, old and tight. It feels like an enemy rather than the good friend it should be. Body Maintenance is the best way to begin a long-lasting and fruitful relationship with yourself.

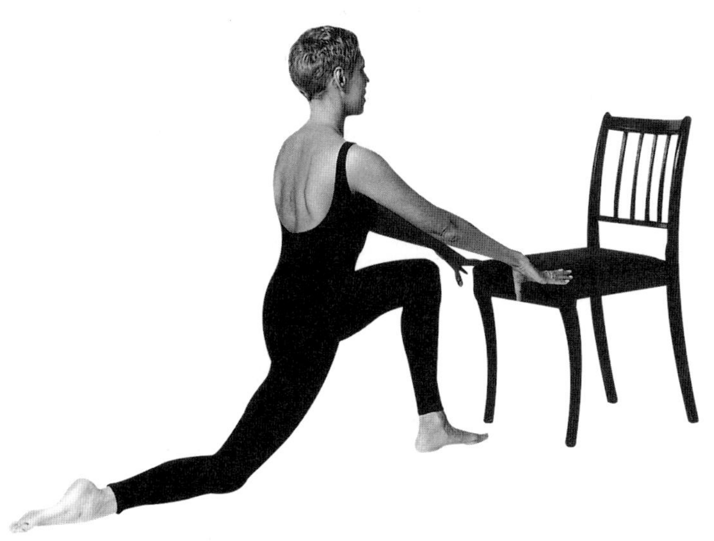

Pilates essentials

Lifestyles can create polarization. In other words, we may go from 'living' at the gym to a total abstinence from any form of exercise, the most common reason being lack of time. I have tried to address this problem by weaving these exercises throughout a busy day, making it easier to implement movement during your free time.

For those of you who have read my first book, *15-Minute Pilates*, many terms and phrases will be readily familiar. The tenets of my Pilates-based Body Maintenance are consistent – although an exercise may change, the principles of the method do not.

10-Step Pilates has been divided into four packages containing exercises, which if done daily and conscientiously, will maximize your energy internally and improve your appearance. You will begin to shed any old unflattering images of yourself as you learn special breathing and visualization techniques which will heighten the effects of each movement. Imagine how you wish to look and you will make it happen.

Talk to dancers, writers, lawyers, just about anyone and you will be told that the most difficult part in any new regime is the beginning. To create the best frame of mind for *10-Step Pilates*, the following concepts are essential.

Breathing

In dance a lot of emphasis is placed on the relationship between breath and movement. However, the importance of breath is a topic rarely addressed in the gym. Pilates differs from conventional forms of exercise in that it concentrates on the correct use of breathing for each and every exercise.

Breath nourishes the body and the brain. People tend to breathe shallowly into their upper bodies when they inhale, into the upper chest and not right down into their lower lobes. If you are breathing deeply, you're working from the inside out. You are energizing and replenishing large areas of your body. Again, it is as much a spiritual as a physical idea.

For most of the exercises in *10-Step Pilates*, you will breathe out on the point of effort. During the exercises you want to think about oxygen as a rejuvenating life-force. Always exhale on the point of effort. If you have a tight area, try and breathe into that – breath is another form of liberation, working from the inside out.

Most people are stronger on one side than on the other, looser on one side and tighter on the other. You are using exercise and breath to create equilibrium in the body.

Control

All the exercises in *10-Step Pilates* are controlled. In this particular instance the word 'controlled' means that the correct body parts are being used. Many people, for example, thinking that they are using their abdominals during an exercise, are, in fact using their bones or hip flexes. Thus, the muscles that should be targeted are not being worked in an efficient way.

Control and precision go together. All exercises for *10-Step Pilates* are done slowly, in a meditative fashion. You focus the mind on what you're doing, you don't allow the mind to wander. You use breath, coordination, control and precision to do a limited number of repetitions well.

You minimize the stress and involvement of other parts of the body. It's preferable to do even five repetitions in a slow and regulated way, than to go through hundreds of motions, during which time nothing effective has happened. In the pelvic tilts, you should be able to feel, literally, one vertebra at a time. The fact that you do 10 repetitions in *10-Step Pilates* well is better than doing many repetitions badly.

The easiest way to look at this is to consider a basic abdominal curl. You will see people contracting their gluteus (the muscles in the buttock) and using their hip flexes rather than using their abdominal muscles. It is *very* easy to find your *Rectus Abdominus* (the upper stomach). It is not difficult to find the upper abdominal muscles. It is much harder to find the lower abdominal muscles located between the navel and the pubic bone. If you constantly use your legs, they will be doing more work than your stomach, which is not the goal of the exercise. Therefore you would have to do many more repetitions to achieve the same effect, had you been working the abdominal muscles properly.

The same principle applies when you are using free-standing weights. In this case, you should be thinking about using internal resistance rather than using your shoulders or snapping your elbows as you use the weights. Focus on the muscles you're using, while making sure that the rest of the body is relaxed and aligned. People often make what is a simple exercise into something quite tortuous, thus creating distortion, tension and the inability to minimize the movements of other parts of their bodies.

Centring

All exercises in *10-Step Pilates* stem from a strong centre which is why, in my studio classes, exercise is taught from the centre. When doing Pilates you work from a strong core. Everything else – your arms, legs and head – are appendages, coming away from the centre. If you have a strong centre, consisting of the abdominal muscles and the whole corset area of the abdomen and lower back – then anything you do with your arms and legs requires much less effort because of that central stability.

The centre is the core of the body. You should think of it as a natural corset. People who have back problems are often put into a corset to re-create the abdominal and back muscles, which support your spine and internal organs. Without those strong muscles you end up with all sorts of problems associated with a weak stomach and back. Many people suffer from backache, which could be alleviated.

Coordination

Children run naturally, but for most adults basic coordination is a major problem. Many people when starting Body Maintenance complain to me, 'I can't coordinate my breath and the movement. It's too much. I've got to concentrate too hard. I can't do it.' Most of us have lost the ability to coordinate the mind and body into a working machine. We no longer have the sense of our feet being in contact with the earth. We've lost the feeling of the way the breath moves naturally through the body. The aim is to retrain the neuromuscular connection between the brain and the body.

This is best illustrated when I try and teach foot exercises to people. I sometimes joke that the feet are very far from the brain and they won't obey, as they haven't been asked to do anything for a long time. Observe people who have lost the use of their hands. They can do the same things with their feet that we can do with our hands. We all have that capability, but we don't employ it. If you don't avail yourself of something it atrophies. Therefore, if you don't use coordination in the physical sense you lose the ability.

Some of the exercises in *10-Step Pilates* appear quite complicated; that's because they're based upon the introduction of a more complicated concept as opposed to mere physical movement. They are trying to reintroduce the mind to the mind/body equation. If I ask my opposite arm and leg to do something at the same time, coordinating from the breath and a strong centre, I should be able to achieve it. If I slip in the street, I am more likely to regain my balance than not. If someone throws a bunch of keys at me, I will probably be able to catch them. Because I have the neuromuscular connection between the mind and body parts, I can be spontaneous, and this is where the proprioceptive concept – the linking of mind and body – comes into play.

In *10-Step Pilates*, we try to re-create your body as a coordinated whole, rather than thinking 'I am exercising an arm or leg or the stomach.' Coordination is paramount to the way the exercises flow. You might see a Pilates exercise that is similar to those used in aerobic classes or at a gym, but the difference between a Pilates exercise and an aerobic one is that, in Pilates, the movement is concentrated exercise and requires minimal effort from other parts of the body.

Postural Realignment

We create stresses and imbalances in our bodies from very early on. People have a tendency to create their own boundaries and limitations. In *10-Step Pilates* you attempt to reconstruct an anatomically correct body in which you feel comfortable.

Most posture is habitual – it is learned, not inherited. Obviously there are some postural disorders that are difficult to correct. There are many people who have scoliosis – a curvature in the spine – and other back disorders, but little of it is congenital. Virtually no one has a 'straight' spine. Everyone tends to have curves to a minimal degree, but it is only through over-using the strong areas and under-using the weak ones that a minor problem can turn into a major one. Then a minimal imbalance becomes uncomfortable and develops into real pain.

Postural realignment is about trying to re-create a body that has reversed these stresses and strains.

Another aspect to postural realignment are injuries incurred as a result of accidents. Sometimes people have to undergo spinal surgery. Even after invasive surgery, a lot of work can be done with the correct use of exercise to re-create a strong, active and functioning body.

Visualization

After people learn the exercises, the next important step is visualization. Visualize the body you want to have for yourself. Visualize the way you want to walk, stand. Direct your energy to these ends.

In *10-Step Pilates* visualization is integral to the process. If you visualize the grounding down through the feet into the earth and the release of the head into the clouds, you can use stretching and mobilization, as well as strengthening exercises, to release a stored up negative self-image. In many of the exercises it is useful to think of energy as a cyclical flow – you are releasing energy and then replenishing it and bringing it back into the body through the use of breath. In a cat stretch, you use breath to create both energy and oxygen so as to liberate the tension through each vertebra in the back and to replenish the blood flowing into the discs as a cyclical, life-force-rejuvenating spiral.

These physical exercises can have a huge impact on mental attitudes. Through proper use of visualization, these exercises should have a prolonged effect as they are successfully integrated throughout the day on a step-by-step basis. Soon enough this will become second nature to the way your body reconstructs itself. Think of your goals, feel the transformation as it occurs. This should be seen as an achievement, not a chore. In his own studio, when he was working with injured dancers, Josef Pilates often quoted the 18th-century German philosopher and poet Friedrich von Schiller: 'It is the mind that shapes the body.' Direct the mind and the body will follow.

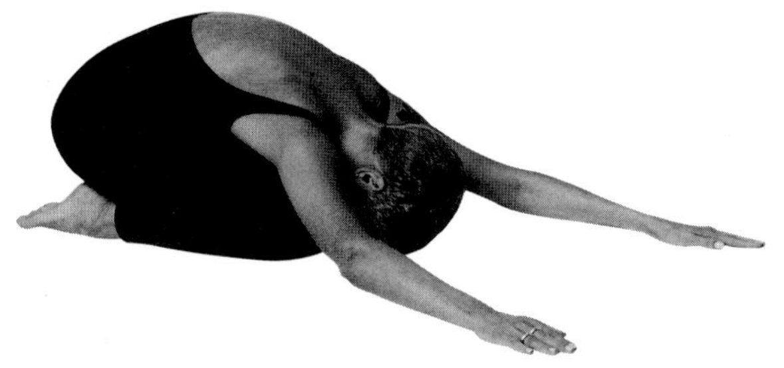

A Dancer's life

by Thomas Paton

I came into dance in a roundabout way. I started taking Latin and Ballroom dancing lessons when I was four, tap and modern dancing when I was four-and-a-half, and then ballet when I was 14 – that's considered very late. I went to a Theatre Arts college where there was a very broad scope of dance styles and techniques, and they encouraged me in the classical field. I left college after three years with some very high dance qualifications. I did a touring production of *West Side Story* straight away and then, having previously auditioned for the London City Ballet, now known as the City of London Ballet, I re-auditioned and was accepted – basically to carry a spear.

However, the choreographer from Paris, Patrice Bart, needed two more male dancers for the *corps de ballet*. Therefore, another spear carrier and myself were chosen to do some actual dancing. I was very lucky. Being able to learn quickly, my technique advanced to that professional company standard. I was 20 years old.

Injury

During my first year in the company, a stress fracture developed on the front of my shin. Any number of bones can be affected by stress fractures. You can get them in your feet, your back, almost anywhere. As a result of the stress and strain the bone starts to crack apart like a fracture.

Basically mine developed as a result of travelling around the country – at times non-stop, occasionally performing in two venues a week, doing one venue for a week and then having two weeks of rehearsals and going back out on the road. We would dance on very steep raked stages – where the stage slopes – and then we'd dance on flat stages. We were performing *Swan Lake* five times a week and then a triple bill at the end of the week for three shows.

I was also given a lot of character dancing in the Russian tradition, having to wear boots and Cossack hats. This required many little jumps as well as sitting on my haunches and kicking my legs up. I had done character dancing at college. In every classical ballet there are *divertimenti* from around the world to entertain the audience, and I was always a

Russian. But my body didn't really like it. Then suddenly, without warning, it was becoming really painful to dance.

Dancers are used to some small injury, some niggly little problem, an ache or pain, as when you're on tour you tend to be tired, but you still have to go out and give a performance. Dancers think whatever the problem is, it will be all right because they're used to pushing through some sort of pain. Also, if you take an evening off, you feel sorry for your friends as they will be forced to share your workload. Instead of taking a break after three acts they might have to go on for a fourth. When on tour, there are only a certain number of dancers and if people leave because of injury, those scheduled for that rare night off have to work.

Eventually, the pain became excruciating and I was forced to stop dancing altogether. I went to the Remedial Dance Clinic, where I did Pilates for the first time for a period of eight weeks. Subsequently, my second year with the London City Ballet went smoothly, and I was sure that my stress fracture was gone for good.

Birmingham Royal Ballet

I then got a job at Sadler's Wells, the touring company of the Royal Ballet at the time the company relocated to Birmingham. For the most part my daily schedule was as follows: an hour-and-a-half class at 10.30 am, followed by a 15-minute break and then into rehearsals until one. At two, back for more rehearsals until 5.30. After two free hours, we had dinner and then back to the theatre for costume, make-up and warm-up for a performance, which finished at 10.30 at night. Afterwards to bed and up the next day for class at 10.30 in the morning.

Some people presume that professional ballet dancers come in at 7.25 in the evening, put on costume and make-up, go on stage, and just dance ... Then they get to go home and have a life, but that's far from the truth, especially on tour.

Almost immediately after I joined Sadler's Wells, more character work came into the repertory. That had been a contributing factor towards my stress fracture in the first place. Once I went back to doing those Russian cossack jumps, my shin just couldn't cope.

Body Maintenance

I had already met Lesley Ackland, the Remedial Dance Consultant for the Birmingham Royal Ballet, who had set up a small but efficient Pilates suite for the company. Before my injury – because of my previous experience with Pilates – I made use of the equipment, which included a plié machine or 'Reformer' – a bed that you lie on with springs and pulleys attached so you do all the exercises as if you are standing on the floor – a 'Cadillac' or 'Four-Poster' – a large bed, again with springs and pulleys attached to it, which is much more of a mat work-based bed – and a sloping bed for stretching. The suite also had weights and mats for floor work.

After my injury I probably should have worn a plaster cast at the onset, and I might not have been off for quite as long as I was, but I was averse to having one. Therefore, I was on crutches to reduce the weight bearing on the injured shin. Eventually it was decided that I should return to London and start intensive rehabilitation.

For four months Lesley and I worked for three or four hours a day in the Body Maintenance Studio at Pineapple, in Covent Garden. The exercises for my stomach were done with my knees bent over a box. I did everything from a sitting or kneeling position, or on my back so that no stress would go down through my right femur. I even did ankle weights with the weight strapped around my knee.

Changing Body Shape

In the course of doing Pilates, my body shape – my physicality – changed three times. When I wasn't doing a lot of weight-bearing exercises with my lower legs, I was able to strengthen up my upper body. Everything lengthened out, but as soon as I resumed dancing I slimmed down a bit. Then it was time to look at my legs and observe how I was re-adjusting the muscle balance, not to a different ballet technique but applying them to ballet technique in general, and using modification so as to avoid future injury.

Now every year since I've done some kind of character dancing I've never had a problem. For me, the key to Pilates is change. Being able to

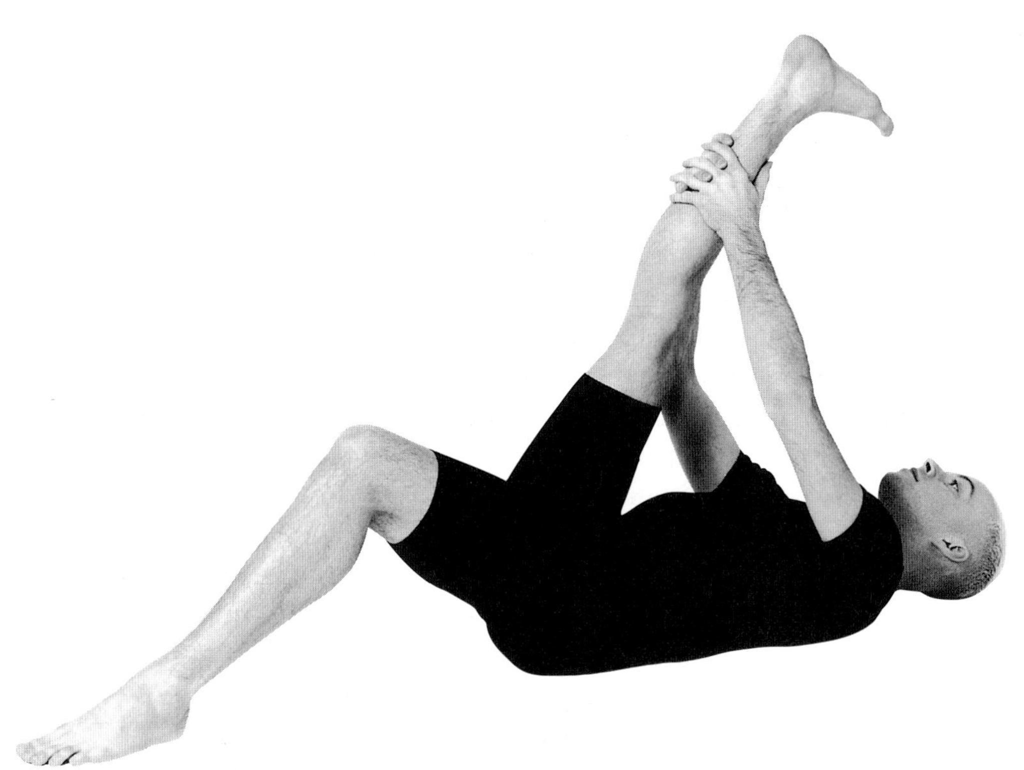

look at your body, note the progression and after six months think, 'there's nothing wrong with the exercise, but what should I be doing to get even more from it?' That's where Lesley and the Body Maintenance Studio play a vital role. She continually tailors the exercises specifically to my needs.

My main problem was a weak centre, and a very mobile but weak lower back as a consequence of doing ballroom dancing all those years ago. Therefore, we concentrated on building up a strong centre to stabilize my centre of gravity, to make certain that my bodyweight was in the right place. If your bodyweight is too far back on your feet, you then put pressure through the front of your legs. The sheath muscles rub on the front of the shin. That creates tension and then the bone starts to stress.

Pilates also helped me make decisions more quickly when I was dancing, and enabled me to compensate for the little mistakes. The neuromuscular connection that Lesley talks about occurred in my performance. Instead of a teacher telling me where to be and how to dance, I was able to make certain decisions for myself. I could accommodate for things that inevitably happen during live performance, such as someone not being in the right place, or breaking my shoe. Pilates has given me an edge, in that I can adjust my body without even thinking about it. If a dancer is pirouetting and not on his centre, he falls off. With the exercises I was doing, I was able to adjust my body and stay on my centre until the end of the phrase. That's the difference between Pilates and other exercise. If you go to the gym, you tell your muscles to do one thing. Alternatively, when you practise Pilates you're encouraging your muscles to work with each other.

The Importance of Pilates to Non-Dancers

My Dad has multiple sclerosis and my Mum has osteoporosis. They live in a small town outside Glasgow, where there is very little physiotherapy. My Dad sees someone once every two weeks. The very little money allotted for health care has to be spread amongst a large number of people. I've shown my parents some Pilates exercises which help them. I'm always aware of their illnesses, but Pilates is extremely gentle. Their few minutes of Pilates a day helps them in their goal of staying healthier for longer.

Some people think if they can't afford to join a gym or can't go to a Pilates studio then they have no chance to improve their fitness level, which is totally wrong. In the beginning it's not how much you do or where you do it, but how much you pay attention to detail, wherever you exercise. In Pilates, less is always more. You have to be sure that you are breathing properly, as well as performing the exercise movements correctly.

It's also so important to take some time for yourself, to calm down, and this is what *10-Step Pilates* is all about. Take those 10 minutes, do the exercises and slow down. I've written about centring myself as a dancer, and that's a physical state, but anyone can centre themselves during their day using breath and exercise.

Pilates won't give you a dancer's body in 10 minutes, but it will give you the best body that you can achieve personally. You're also going to feel better about yourself and more confident with your body. With Pilates, everybody realizes the best version of their body that they can realistically have.

Triple Threat

In my current work in London's West End, I'm considered a 'triple threat'. It's an old Broadway term for someone who is an actor, singer and dancer to an equally high standard. Compared to ballet, musical theatre is a different kind of life. Once a show is set up you might have one 'clean-up call' every few weeks, and if you understudy a role you have one rehearsal every week, so it's much easier in terms of the time you have for yourself. However it is still arduous because it's eight performances a week, for as long as the show runs. I've been in many shows – *Grease*, *Scrooge* and, for the last two years, *Beauty and the Beast*. I performed the principal role of Mr Mistoffelges in *Cats*. During a two-year run I only had eight days off, and those were non-dance technique related injuries. In the first instance, someone tripped me up on a piece of set, and in the second there was some water on the stage and I slipped and fell. In the last five years my shin has not bothered me once, and this is all due to Pilates.

It's very hard for people to accept the fact that they're not going to do a 10-minute step class. They're not going to do 300 sit-ups and sweat. Pilates starts off very slowly and gently, and when you grasp the basic concepts you might not think you're doing a lot at the time, but you're getting your body to work with your brain and all the muscles to connect with each other. Once you make that connection you can do it 10 minutes a day or an hour and a half a day. With the correct approach and only 10 minutes of concentration and an understanding of the technique, many people find that even when their lives are too busy to exercise at all, when they do have just 10 minutes to continue again, their bodies have their own set of physical memories of the exercises and are ready to pick up where they left off, as opposed to starting all over again. For dancers and non-dancers alike, there can be no better promise than that.

Before exercising

Clothes

Ideally you should wear comfortable clothing for exercising, such as leggings, shorts and a T-shirt, or leotard top. Don't wear anything that restricts your movements. Natural fibres such as cotton are best because they are cooler. You can exercise wearing socks or in bare feet. If you are worried about slipping, put on a pair of trainers. Take off any jewellery which might get in the way.

Preparation

Before you start exercising, check the floor for any sharp objects or stray pins. Most of the exercises in *10-Step Pilates* require little or no equipment. However, it is essential to work on a padded surface or a mat. This will protect your spine and prevent any bruising against a hard floor. It is probably worth investing in a proper sports mat. Alternatively you can work on a folded, synthetic blanket, approximately 5 or 6 feet (1.5 to 1.8 metres) long and 1 foot (30 cm) wide. Some exercises involve the use of props like a chair, or a Dynaband (a long piece of elasticized rubber used by physiotherapists, which can be obtained through most health and fitness shops) tied to a stair banister or door handle. Always make sure these are secure. Try exercising in front of a full-length mirror. This will allow you to check exactly what you're doing.

Continue to add exercises daily, depending on how comfortable you feel. Trust your own judgement. If you're unsure, do the pelvic tilts and abdominal exercises (see particularly Steps 1, 5 and 9), then add to them. If you feel any discomfort in your back during an exercise, you still have insufficient core strength to do it. This will change as you gradually build your core strength by doing the other exercises.

Basic Pilates Safety Rules

- Carefully read all the instructions and pay particular attention to the directions for breathing in the exercises.
- Stretch after the relevant strengthening exercises.
- Increase the number of repetitions gradually.
- Stop if you feel nauseous, fatigued or out of breath.
- Seek medical help immediately if you have any chest pains, especially accompanied by pain in the arms, neck, shoulders and/or jaw.
- Check with your doctor if exercising leaves you unnaturally tired.
- Do not overwork the neck, which is a sensitive part of the body. If you cannot remember if you've done the exercises involving this area of the body, it's preferable not to do any more repetitions.
- Hold on to something for support when doing the balancing exercises.
- Stop if you experience back pain or if your muscles start to shake.
- Drink plenty of fluids afterwards, especially when the weather is hot.

Health Advice

It's always a good idea to consult your doctor before embarking on any new exercise programme. If you are over 40 or have not been exercising regularly, a check-up is strongly recommended. Seek the advice of a specialist if you have a known medical condition, any chronic joint problems or are pregnant.

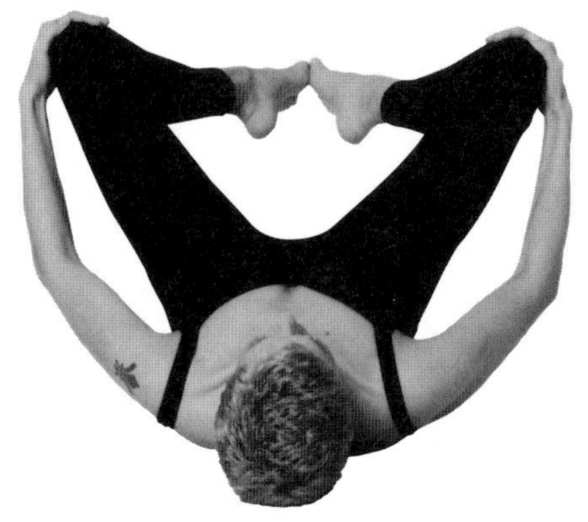

Step 1

Morning energizer

Sleep is supposed to restore us; it is the time when the body regenerates itself. Despite its obviously therapeutic uses, some people don't sleep terribly well. They may have disturbed slumber or they sleep in uncomfortable positions.

Often people wake up feeling lethargic, tight and tense. These exercises focus on limbering and release, and will enable you to start your day in a positive frame of mind. These gentle mobilizing exercises early in the day will reconstruct some of the body's internal alignment. This group of six exercises will wake you up, stimulate you and get your joints moving. They will also initiate the feeling of alignment – of standing up straight, feeling balanced and positive.

Exercise Mat or Towel

In all the exercises which involve lying on the floor, it is recommended that you use an exercise mat, but a large bath towel will do. Don't do these exercises on a wooden floor with only a towel. A bath towel placed on a carpet should give enough support to your spine.

Concentrating on limbering and release, this 10-minute programme of morning stretches focuses on releasing the lower spine, hips and gently loosening the upper body. The spine, the upper and lower back and the muscles in the backs of your leg, the hamstrings, will be released. One movement, based on a classic Pilates exercise, opens up your spine and releases through your discs. Hip rotations will lubricate your hips. The arm exercises will open your shoulder girdle and start getting you to focus on breathing. Finally, there is a side stretch done with a towel to generally stretch and open up. After the Morning Energizer you want to feel physical liberation and a spiritual awaking.

Exercise 1.

Rolling Up Like a Ball

This exercise can be difficult; work your way into it. Sit holding on to your shins. From photograph 1, you can see that I'm curled up like a ball. As you breathe out you roll backwards, and as you breathe in you roll up to a seated position.

1

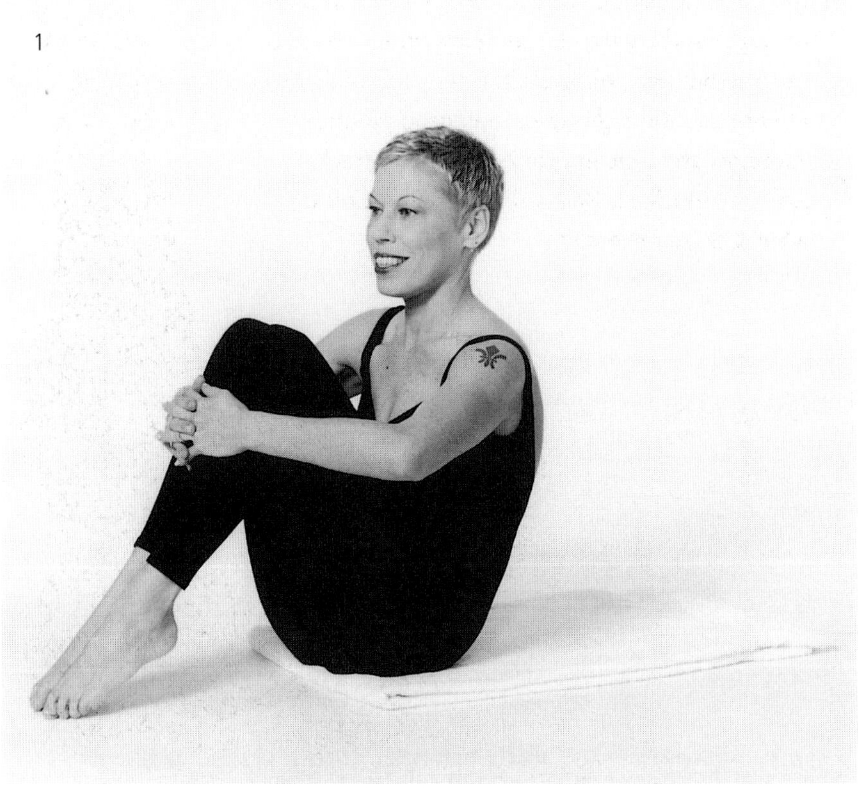

WATCHPOINT

Don't roll too far back onto your neck.

Many people don't have a lot of flexibility in the spine, so you might have a problem in getting back up. If this is the case, come back up normally and start the roll again.

Keep the heels close to your bottom all the way through, and try to relax your shoulders. As you breathe out and roll back, the stomach pulls in. Do not roll too high up on the neck. All the exercises are done approximately 10 times. Rolling Up Like a Ball is the exercise I first do when I myself exercise.

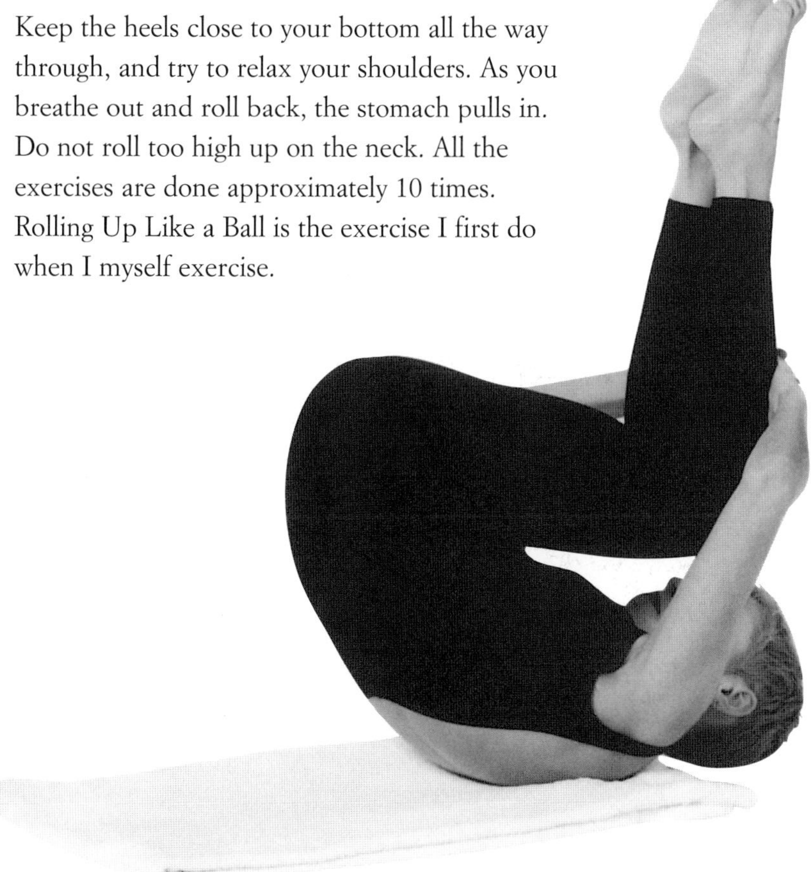

2

Exercise 2.
Hip Mobility Exercise

As we get older the hips get tighter, and there is less articulation in the hip socket.

Lie on a large towel or an exercise mat. The feet are together and you are basically holding on just below the knees. If you feel uncomfortable, put a towel behind your head. The body should not move, the head is resting.

1

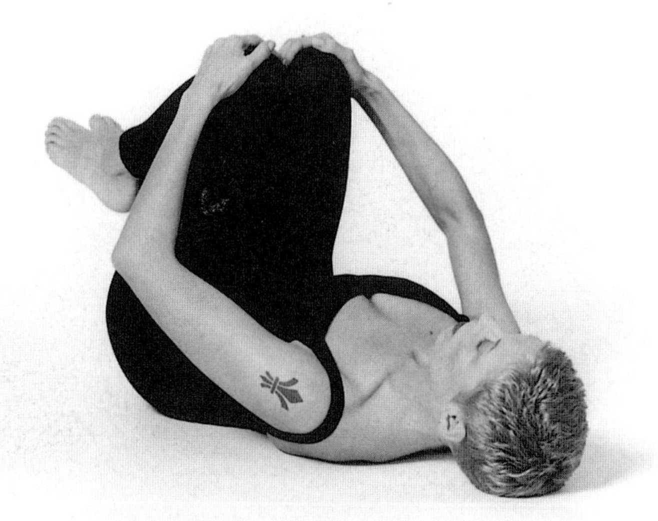

Holding on below the knees, toes together, you rotate your hips 10 times in one direction and 10 times in the other, to lubricate your hips.

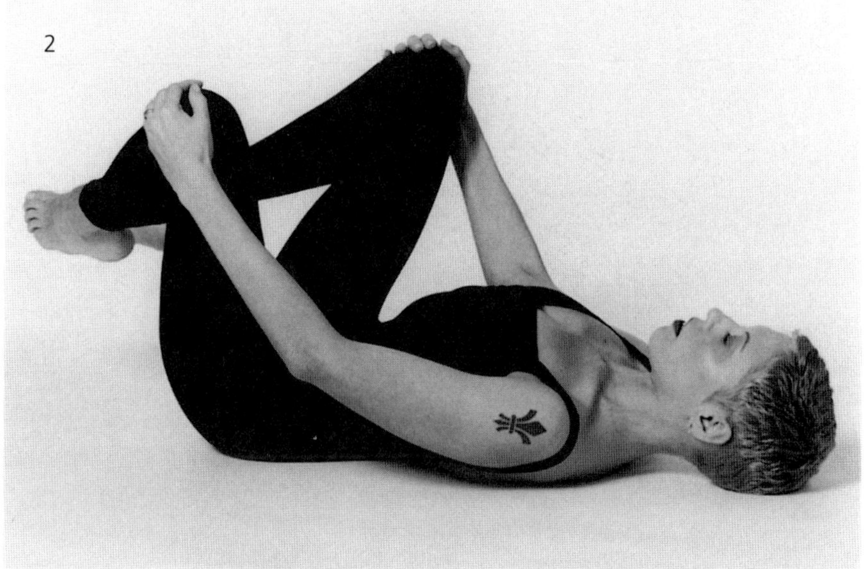

WATCHPOINT

You hold on to your shins and thighs, never the knees.

Hip Mobility Exercise (cont.)

Keeping the toes together, start with the knees apart. As you breathe normally, they come into the chest, they then open and come around. It doesn't matter in which direction you go. This exercise will also help to warm your lumbar spine and the entire pelvis area. You may feel a gentle stretch in your inside thighs, if they're tight. Don't force this feeling of stretch. Just feel the mobilization. You're getting blood to flow through your hips and releasing tension through your pelvis. Don't have the legs too far away from you. Keep the knees over the hips. Your legs do not hang off your body. Your tailbone is heavy and supported by the mat or towel at all times.

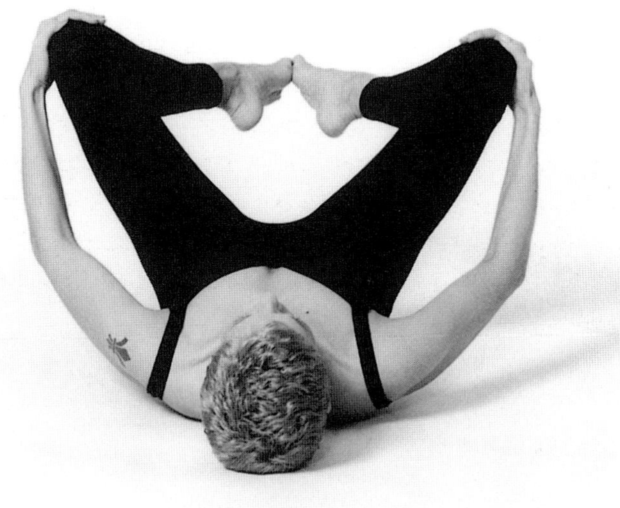

Exercise 3.
Full-Body Wake-Up Stretch

Lie on your back with a towel behind your head and flex your feet – your toes pointing up towards your knees – hold your hands, fingers entwined. As you breathe in, the elbows bend so the hands almost touch the crown of the head.

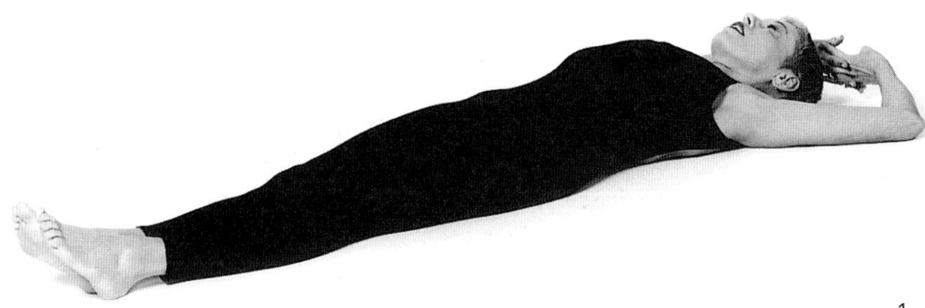

1

As you breathe out, stretch your arms as far away from you as you can, flex your feet and stretch. Breathe in, bend your elbows, relax, breathe out and stretch. You'll feel this stretch in the back of your legs, your hamstrings, your calf muscles, feet and shoulders. You may feel a stomach stretch as well.

Do approximately 10 repetitions.

You can either do this exercise with the hands crossed or the fingers interlaced. Breathe in, breathe out, and stretch. As you breathe out and stretch, the shoulders shrug up towards the ears. As you breathe in, relax the shoulders, and let them drop. The hands come towards the crown of your head or forehead, the legs relax. As you breathe out, the fingers and hands stretch away, the shoulders lift, the feet stretch towards the other end of the room with flexed feet. The body is stretched and energized.

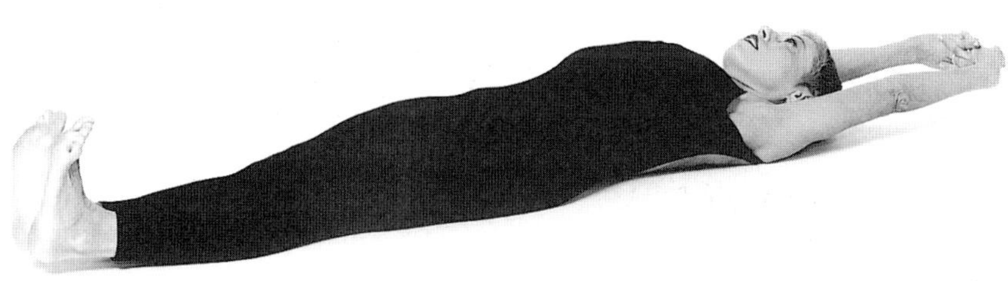

2

Exercises 4 & 5.

Warm-Ups for Shoulders and Back

These two exercises are about postural awareness. At this point do not stand on a towel unless you feel very secure. This exercise is better done with bare feet, so you can feel the contact with the floor.

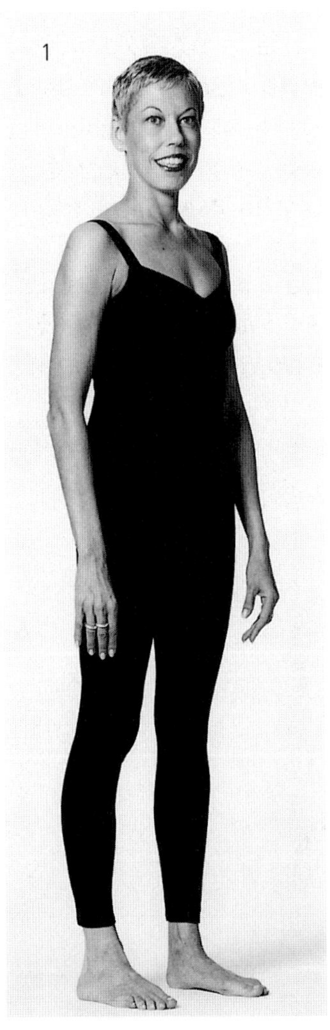

Stand with your feet hip-width apart. Relax your feet. Make sure the weight is evenly placed over your feet, try not to sink either forward or backward. The toes are relaxed and lengthened as if they're softening into sand. When you're standing upright the stomach is gently pulled in, the tailbone drops, the pelvis is in neutral. You're not gripping your hamstrings or the back or front of your legs.

Start with the arms naturally relaxed at your side. They don't hang behind you, they gently soften, as if your middle finger is stretching down the outside of your thigh, lengthening away. In this position the hands are just in front of you. The shoulders are relaxed and the head is in a neutral position. Don't let your head drop forward or back. Let it sit on top of your shoulders. Use visualization techniques and think of your head as a blossom sitting on the stem of a plant. The head is just softly there. The knees are released.

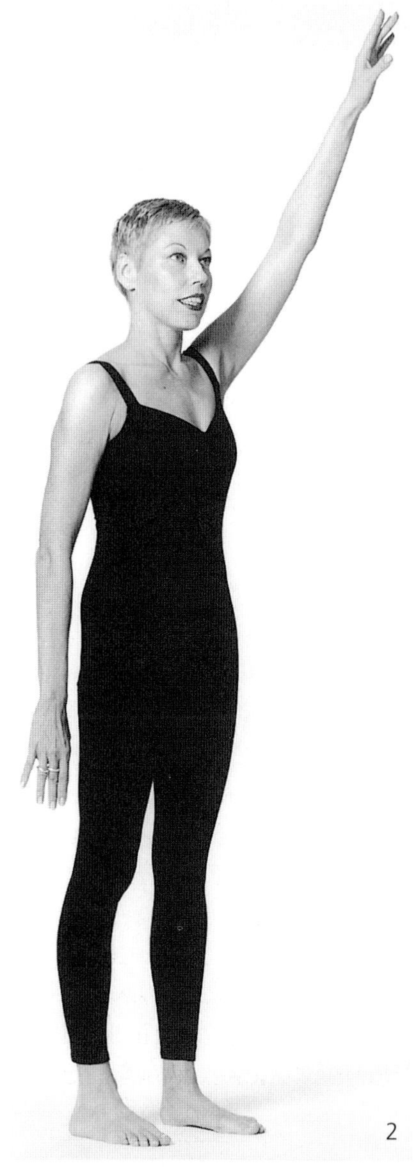
2

The first exercise is very simple. Begin with the arms beside you. As you breathe out, one arm reaches to the ceiling, and the other arm gently reaches to the wall behind you without any shift in the feet, the pelvis, the upper back or the neck. If you're feeling that shift you are taking the movement too far for your initial flexibility. This exercise can be done either 10 times, 5 on each side, or 20, which is 10 on each side, alternating the arms.

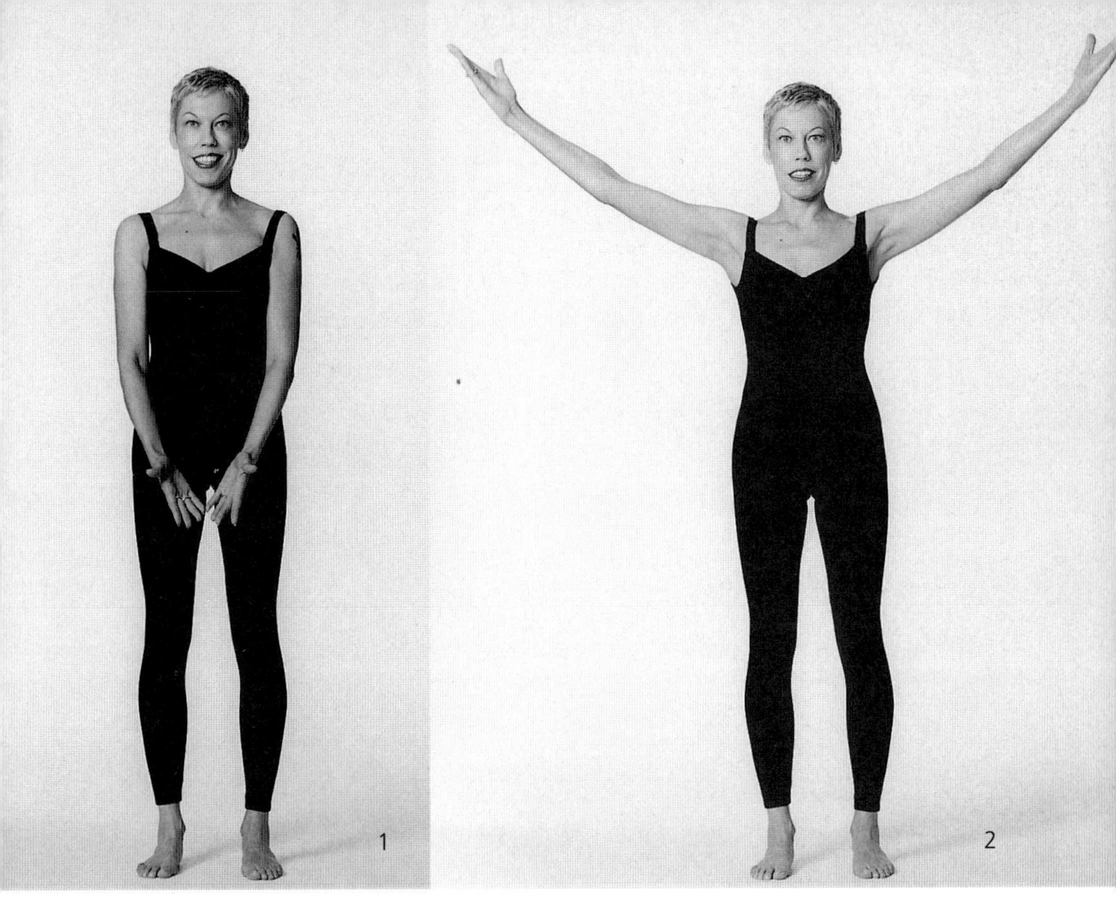

The second exercise targets the same area. Start with the same postural alignment, no gripping of the feet, no tensing of the buttocks – everything is relaxed and calm. Straighten both your arms and bring them in front of you with the tips of the little fingers touching (photograph 1).

As you breathe out you take a slice and reach to the corners of the room. The arms stay straight all the way through. Breathe in, breathe out, then slice, reaching for the corners of the room (photograph 2).

WATCHPOINT

With any of the arm exercises, at no point do you lock your elbows. The joints are in line, the shoulders, the elbows, the wrist, all the fingers – don't break at the wrist.

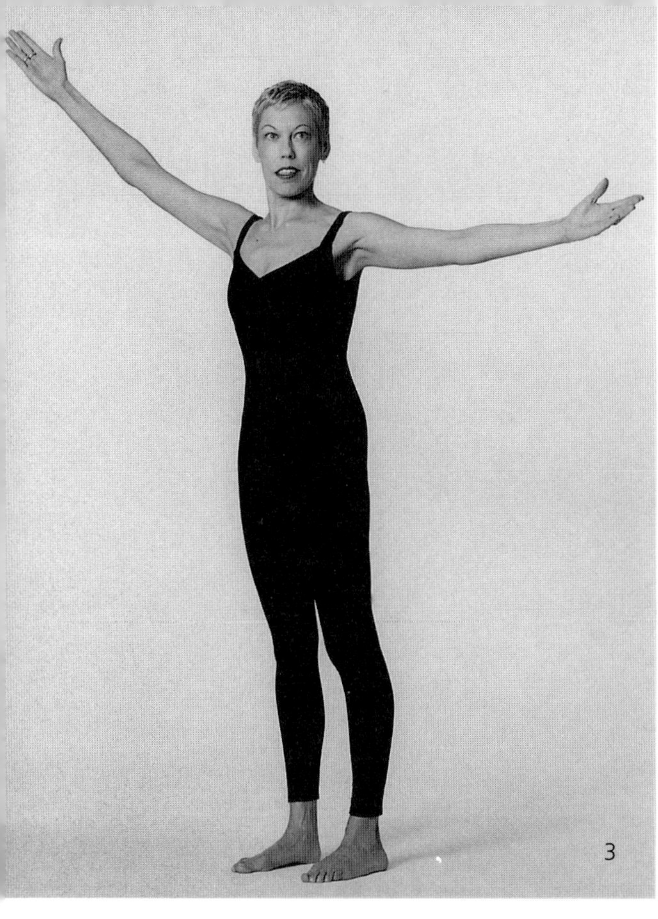

After you've done this second exercise 10 times you may do a few on the diagonal. You slice, gently twist and the head follows. You will feel a gentle stretch across the chest and some stretching through the shoulders.

These exercises are also about coordination. In the first exercise both arms work rhythmically, alternating. In the second exercise you want both arms to start and end at the same point. You don't want one arm to begin before the other.

Exercise 6.
Waist Stretch

Stand in the same position, holding a hand towel nice and wide between your arms. Breathe out, stretch to one side. Breathe in, straighten up, and breathe out to stretch to the other side. Don't lift your shoulders up to your ears, and stretch only as far as you don't shorten on the underneath side.

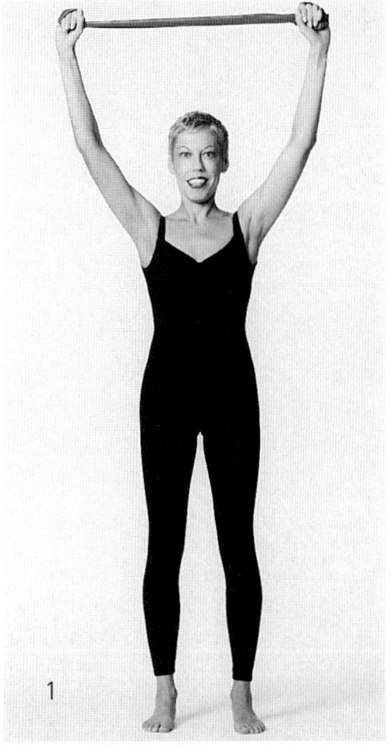
1

Your weight should be evenly balanced over both feet. You'll know you've gone too far if you feel one foot coming off the floor. The weight is over the second toe, as in all of the standing exercises. Hips don't move very much because it is a waist-energizing stretch. Breathe out as you take the stretch, breathe into the centre and breathe out as you change.

Do approximately 10 repetitions on each side.

The Waist Stretch is related to core strength, which will be examined in greater detail later in this book. You engage your abdominals to stabilize your pelvis and your spine during a gentle waist stretch, the body does not collapse from side to side.

WATCHPOINT

Keep the weight evenly distributed over both feet for the duration of the exercise and don't allow yourself to tip from one side to the other.

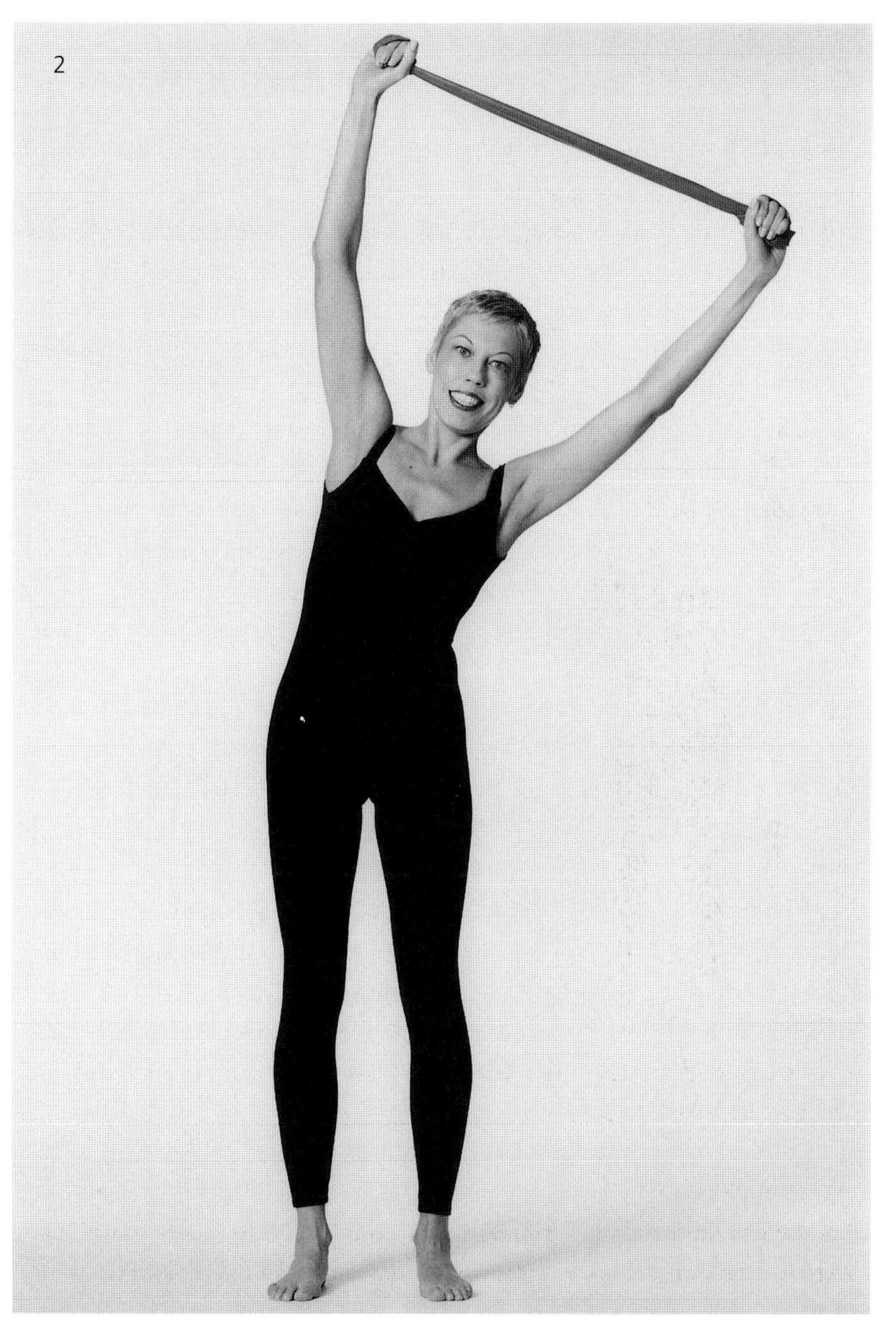
2

Pilates at the airport

Brian Eley, creative director at a London design consultancy, does 15 to 20 minutes of Pilates exercises every morning. 'I always feel that I'm not fully awake or standing erect until I've exercised. It really stretches and relaxes me, and releases my lower back, which I may have twisted during the night.

'I've been going to Lesley Ackland for about 10 years and have been exercising in the morning during all that time. A few of the exercises I can do wherever I am, for instance in hotel rooms or on one occasion in the departure lounge of an airport. I've even done them on the floor at work, if I feel I need a stretch.'

Sciatic Pain

'My problem is with my lower back. When I first started going to Body Maintenance I had regular, very painful "incidents". On one occasion I had to be shipped back from holiday abroad with my back taped up with bandages. Two Christmases in a row were spent laid out flat on the floor with sciatic pain in my legs, even down to my feet.

'I had been to my GP. He'd referred me to physiotherapy, where they simply gave me a corset to wear around my waist. They didn't seem to know how to deal with my back and I wasn't benefiting at all. My wife has always been interested in dance. She heard about Lesley and tried Pilates. When my wife described the class to me, it didn't sound as if I would fit in; Lesley dealt with dancers and performers, not people like me. But when Pilates starts to work you forget about all that.

'My physical trouble seems to be the result of doing no real physical exercise between the ages of 12 and 35. I was healthy but I didn't take regular exercise. I'm tall and skinny, and I would often over-extend or bend or stoop or stand in the wrong way. So I developed really bad posture. When I first started Pilates I was doing very desk-bound work, where I might spend up to twelve hours a day at a desk in front of a computer. Although the work has changed a great deal, it's still office work and rather sedentary. I also travel a lot, and wherever I am I can do Pilates.'

On the Office Floor

'If I'm feeling really bad, a simple hip roll can help. Most of the people whom I've worked with for a long time know I do Pilates. You can work closely with people for years and know nothing about them; some are a little surprised at first to see me rolling around the floor! When I exercised in an airport lounge I didn't care what others thought. You're never going to see those people again. They're all flying off to different parts of the world. Your own well-being comes first.

'I will be doing Pilates for as long as it helps me. Whenever I feel back pain now, it's usually very minor, and I know how to correct my body. I do the appropriate exercise and prevent the pain from developing. With Pilates I can keep myself out of trouble.'

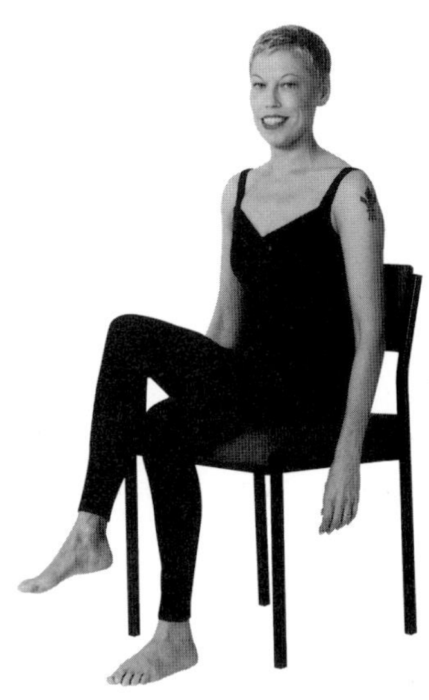

Step 2
Integrated postural awareness at work

With these exercises you will maximize posture and energy levels in environmentally unfriendly conditions. You will learn to sit and stand correctly throughout the day. New habits will form and, once learned, will be hard to break. Your body will feel comfortable and well-balanced, freeing you to be mentally alert.

Generally people sit badly. They sink into their hips when they sit down. Most people are not as active as they should be because of the restrictions in their daily lives. These exercises will take you back to basics, re-creating the way you sit. The emphasis in these exercises is not on complicated movement but on visualization.

You are sitting at your desk, with your chair at the right level, with your feet grounded through the floor, and equal pressure down through both feet. Your lower back is supported in the chair, the upper back floating above with no tension. A shoulder stretch has also been included, which will release tense shoulders. You then breathe into your stomach and, on the exhale, you contract your stomach into the back of the chair, concentrating on feeling that movement of internal support as you grow taller and more confident.

Step 2 also focuses on how you project yourself while sitting at your desk.

Exercise 1.

Sitting Properly

Sit with your back supported by a chair. Your tailbone is heavy, both feet are evenly placed on the floor. You are in contact from your centre directly down through your feet into the floor. You're going to channel your energies from your centre out through the crown of your head. Your shoulders are relaxed, your arms are relaxed because your middle back is supported. Your tailbone will drop and your abdominals will naturally pull back towards your spine. Again, try to think of your head sitting naturally on top of your shoulders, not pushing forward and not pushing back.

WATCHPOINT

If you force your shoulders back and your lower back arches away from the chair, you know your shoulders are still too rounded for you to maintain this position and be anatomically correct.

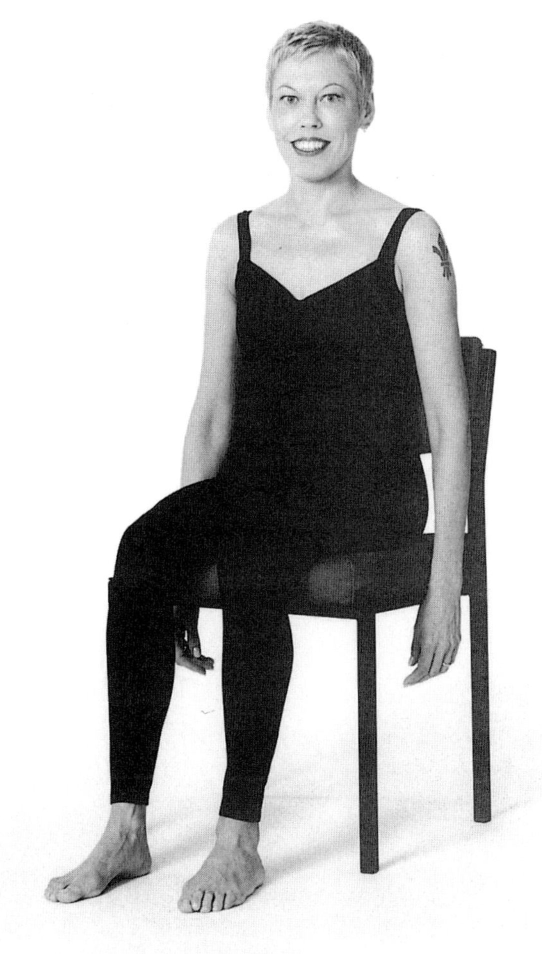

Integrated postural awareness at work

Exercise 2.

Breathing

Starting with this basic seated position, place your fingers on your lower abdominals, the space between your pubic bone and your navel. As you breathe in the stomach gently expands, filling with oxygen. As you breathe out the stomach pulls away from your fingers and settles back into the chair, your navel pulls away from your fingers and you feel the energy going in to support the lower back. Repeat 10 times.

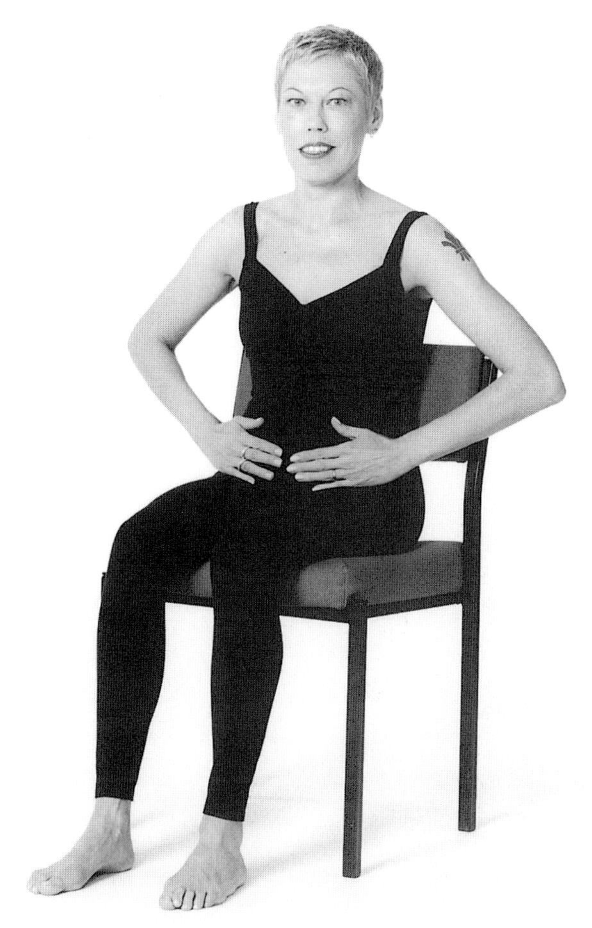

Exercise 3.
Foot Lifts

You can either have your fingers on your abdomen in the same place as the previous exercise or allow your arms to hang naturally beside you. As you breathe in your abdomen gently softens or expands into your fingers, as you breathe out you very gently let one foot float off the floor, feeling the connection of the navel to the spine. Place the foot down, make sure you have even pressure through both feet again and change legs. The coordination is important. Start off Foot Lifts very slowly; eventually you will be able to do them faster so the interchange emanates from a stable pelvis and a strong abdomen.

Initially the change from one leg to the other might feel unstable as you don't have the core strength to coordinate alternate leg lifts automatically. The feet should float off the floor.

10 lifts with each leg, alternating each time.

WATCHPOINT

If you lift your feet too high, you will feel your pelvis sink back into the chair and you'll lose that postural alignment. Your tailbone will tuck underneath and your back will curl.

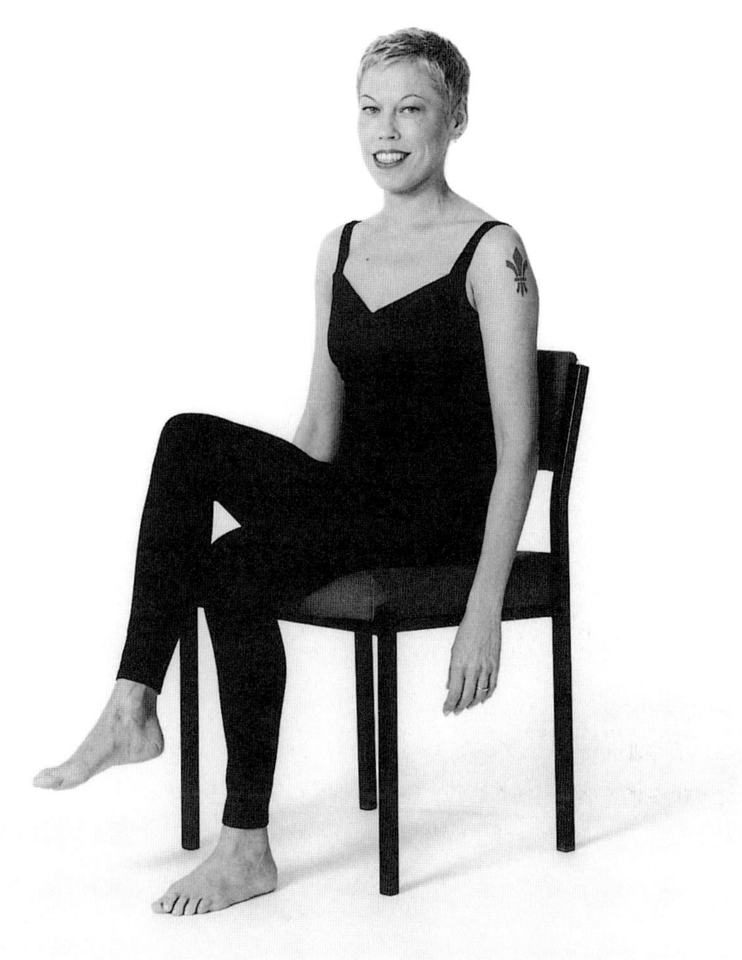

Exercise 4.
Relax Your Ankles

This exercise will relax your ankle, calf and foot, and it will give you a conscious feeling of the connection between your body and the earth.

Slip your shoes off, cross one knee over the other and very gently circle your ankle very slowly, so that you take six seconds to circle the ankle in one direction, approximately six to eight times. Change directions and repeat, then do the same thing with the other ankle.

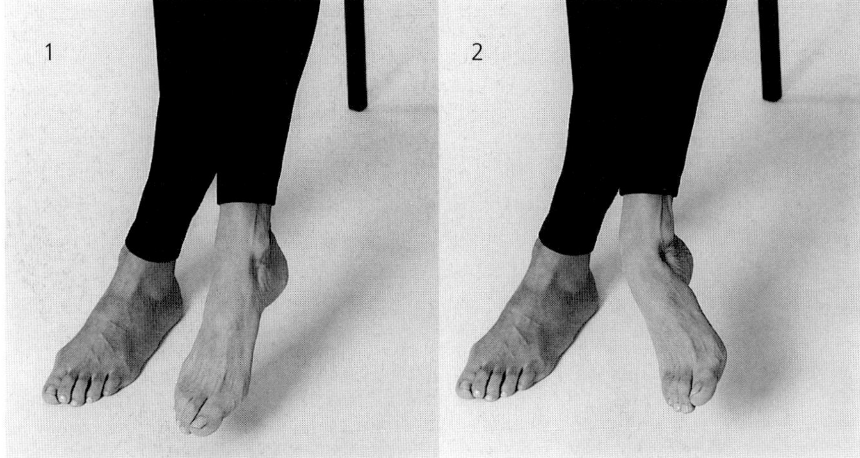

WATCHPOINT

Try to keep your toes relaxed, don't grip with your toes. Do not move the bones in your lower leg – the tibia and fibula. Think of your ankle bones as pebbles that you're gently shaking. As you're circling the ankle, the pebbles are lubricating and relaxing. If you tense your foot and lower leg, this won't happen. Your ankle and calf will feel warmer after this exercise, if completed slowly and rhythmically.

Exercise 5.

Shoulder Stretch

Seated in your chair, all the above rules apply: stomach pulled in, tailbone dropped, both feet evenly balanced on the floor. You think of your energy evenly placed down through both feet. Very gently, take your right hand and place it on your left shoulder blade, palm facing down. Take your other hand and try to reach and connect your fingers behind you. If you can't do this initially, don't worry, aim to. Without arching your back or sticking your chest out, gently open out the right or the left top arm to stretch. Keep the neck long. Do the other side, then approximately five times on each side, alternating sides.

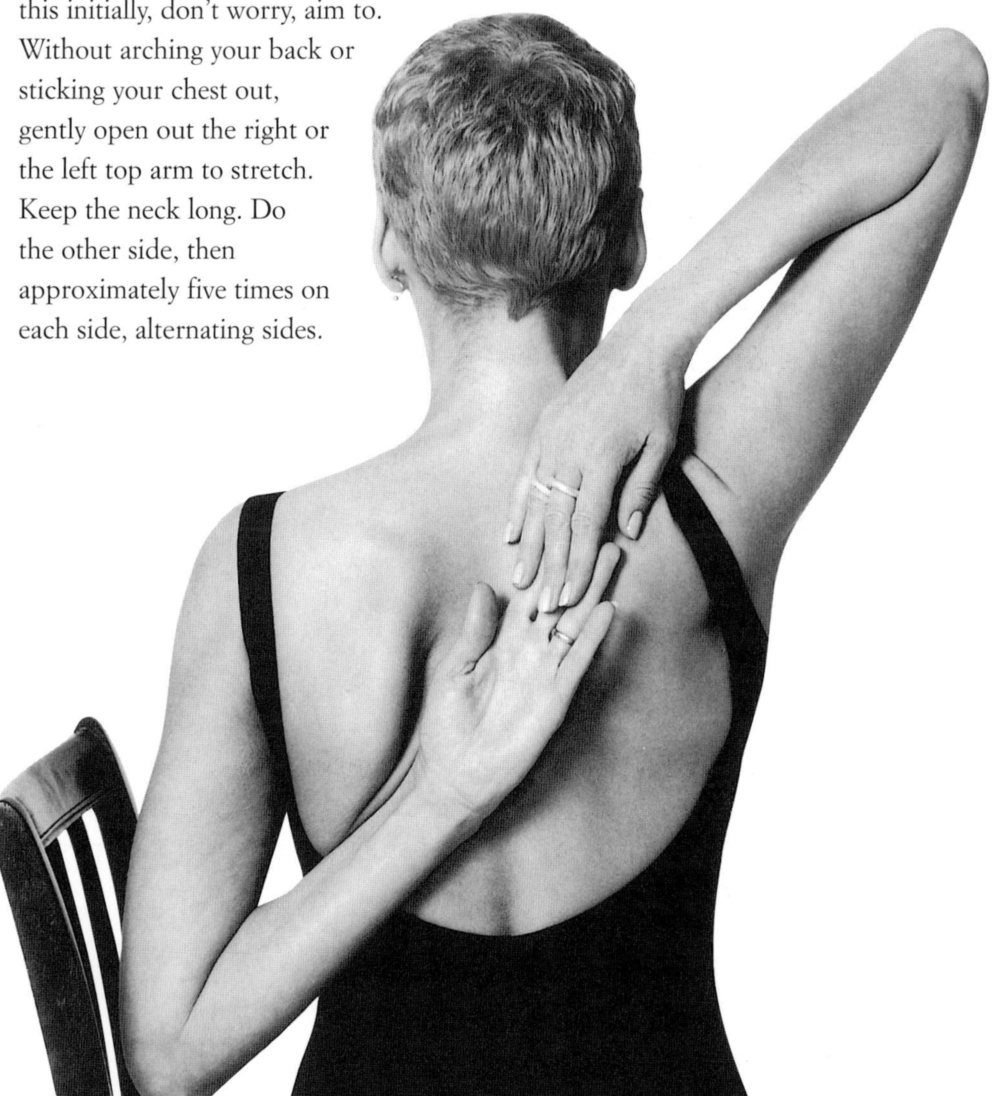

Exercise 6.
Neck Stretch

This Neck Stretch should not be done more than four times.

Sitting in your chair, gently place the palm of your hand not on your neck, but behind the crown of your head.

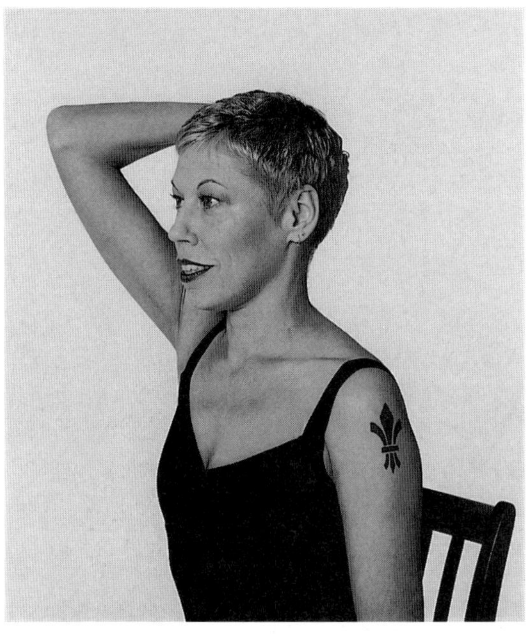

If you're sitting in the right position with your feet comfortably apart, drop your chin towards your chest without leaning forward, look at your big toe and gently press your head against your hand; feel the neck stretching. Hold for 20 seconds. Relax, do the stretch on the left and once more on either side.

WATCHPOINT

Middle back should be supported, tailbone dropped, don't let the chin go forward.

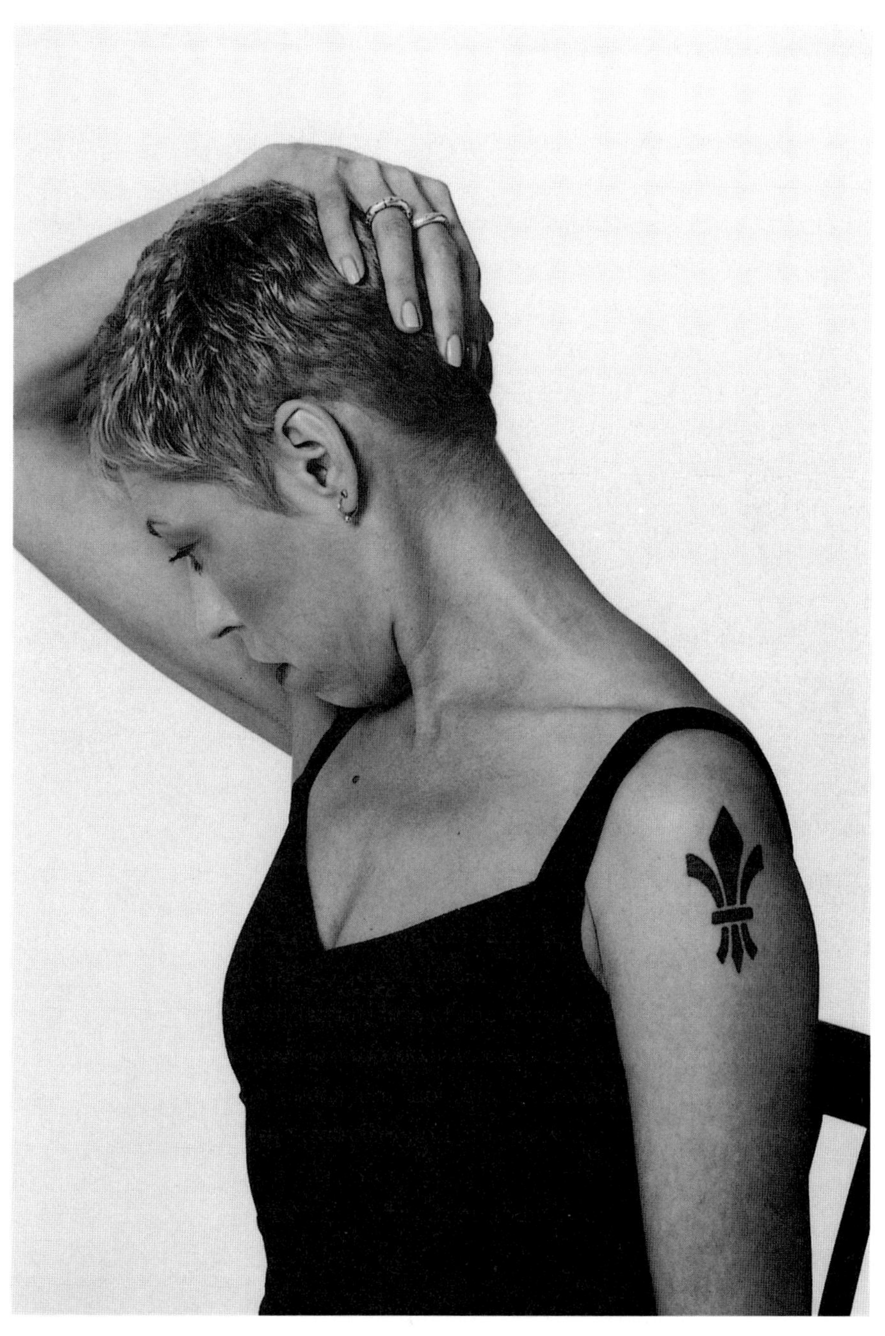

Office posture

Graphic designer Olivia Norton has worked in London for the last eight years. She spends most of her working day sitting in front of a computer. In the past her back had locked by the evening, and she had great difficulty standing up or walking.

'Now I do certain Pilates exercises at my desk. Apparently it's a huge problem for people working at computers. They don't breathe. What happens to me is that at times when I am concentrating intensely on my work I tend to hold my breath. It's really common. I watched a colleague who sits across from me do it. We made a pact that when we have a particularly hard task, we remind each other "Breathe! Breathe!"

'I also suffer from scoliosis and have a bulging disc in my lower back. I don't know how I got the disc problem, but until I started Pilates I was becoming less mobile and weaker and weaker. It was a vicious circle. As I became weaker, I became less able to do things, and more vulnerable.'

Live with Pain

'I had been told by the NHS that I had a chronic back problem and that I would have to learn to live with the pain, or have an operation, which at best might have dubious results.

'I tried Yoga and other forms of exercise but found them "too violent". My back was in pain after exercising. By the time I arrived at the Body Maintenance studio, I had almost given up hope of recovery.

'Lesley said it would take six months until "you're not in pain and another six months to get fit". No one had suggested the pain might go away.

'Admittedly I was nervous in the beginning. I was frightened to do anything. I slowly learned that movement didn't necessarily mean pain. Much of my early work took place on the mat, and focused on strengthening the abdominal muscles. I always returned to the Body Maintenance Studio because I felt immediate relief during and after every class. At first the pain would come perhaps during that same night or the next day, but after a few months it started to diminish for longer periods.'

Gentle Exercise

'Initially I did a few back exercises and they were gentle. Over the years my exercises have changed, becoming stronger and more complicated. Pilates works for a variety of reasons. The breathing centres you and enables you to calmly and methodically focus your attention on your body.

'It has made me more aware of my body and lifestyle. The time one spends doing Pilates turns you on to a frequency where you pay attention to your being in all sorts of ways. You just start to notice what you're doing. In the past I'd be physically very unaware of how I sat at a desk, my legs crossed, one hand twisted around the phone, my other hand on the computer mouse, leaning into the desk. You can do that all day long and not even think about it, and at the end of the day wonder why you're in pain.'

Second Sense

'Pilates is like a second sense. You pay attention to how you sit, walk, and stand. It may sound peculiar but it happens. Even at the best of times people have a tendency to not listen to their bodies. There is a difference between having confidence in Pilates and listening to your own body. Lesley always says "If you're in pain, stop." You are inclined to think "No! Carry on, I must do this exercise. This is good, this is strong. Push through the pain."

'That's absolute nonsense. I have had relapses with Lesley – invariably when I've been overdoing things and feel tired. I used to think, "Rubbish, I am just going to just carry on." But that just makes everything worse. It takes longer to recover and get back to where you were. When you're in pain you have to stop and think, don't be mean to yourself. Don't try to do things you can't, and the end result will be slow, steady progress.

'I went to Derbyshire this weekend and I walked for seven hours both days. I climbed hills, and ran down them. Three years ago I couldn't bend over a sink to brush my teeth, walking gave me sciatica, I couldn't sit down for more than a few minutes without pain! Pilates is wonderful, but it contrasts strongly with the way most of us habitually live.'

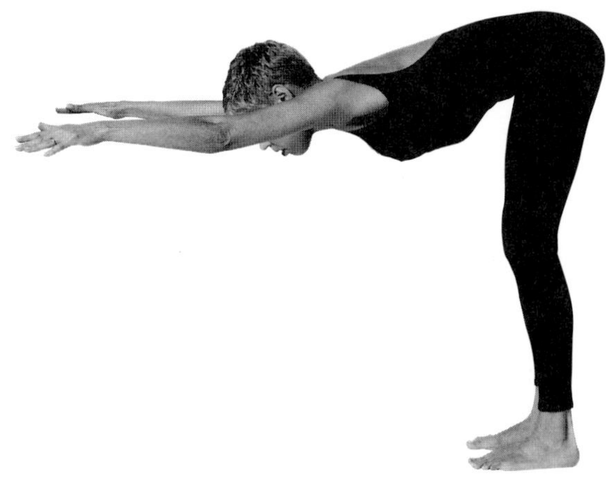

Step 3
Midday break

'Aerobic' is a very general term that can indicate anything from climbing the stairs to taking a short walk. An active aerobic break combined with stretches and body-releasing exercises makes a lunch break a good time to rejuvenate and recharge.

The human mind and body don't function at their best after working for eight consecutive hours. You need to have a space or break in your working day, whether it's a brisk walk or reading a newspaper. A change of environment – physical or mental – will recharge your batteries. Your mind and body will be clearer and you'll feel less sluggish in your working environment.

Step 3 is a restart and refocus. It involves a lot of stretching. It will address the areas that are tight from sitting and working, and will be especially helpful for those who work in front of a computer screen.

You will stand up and do some very simple foot exercises, such as grasping the floor with your toes and releasing, followed by calf stretches, a shoulder stretch and a cat stretch. There is also a stretch in which you stand in the doorway and release your shoulders. This focuses the energy away from the tight, work-induced areas so you can then feel relaxed and liberated when you lunch. You can then enjoy your lunch break, as you will have rid yourself of the work-related muscular stress.

Exercise 1.

Doming

This exercise follows from the beginning of the day exercises in Step 2. Doming is better done with bare feet. Very gently lift your foot so that you're just resting on your heel. As you place your foot on the ground, spread your toes and try to separate them. Ideally they will all spread and separate at the same time. (Imagine doing Doming with your hand, you lift and separate your fingers as you place them down.)

Holding your toes down, you draw up the arch underneath your foot, without gripping your toes. Relax. As you flex onto the heel and spread the toes, imagine having chewing gum under the ball of your foot. You draw – without gripping the floor – your toes up and relax. In the beginning you might get cramp in your foot.

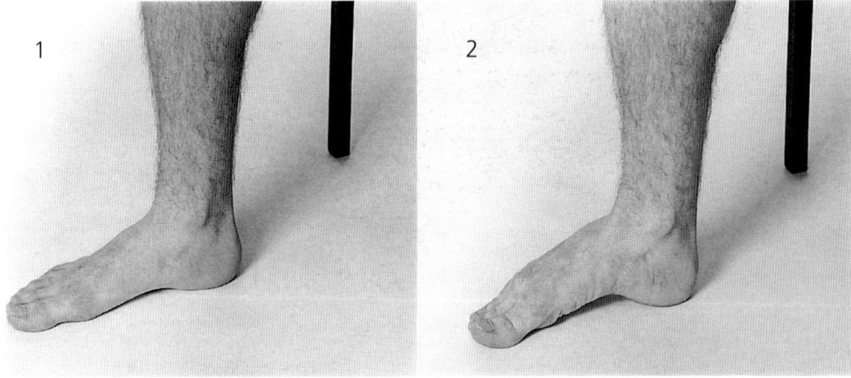

Do 10 repetitions with each foot.

WATCHPOINT

Do not let your toes become 'clawed'.

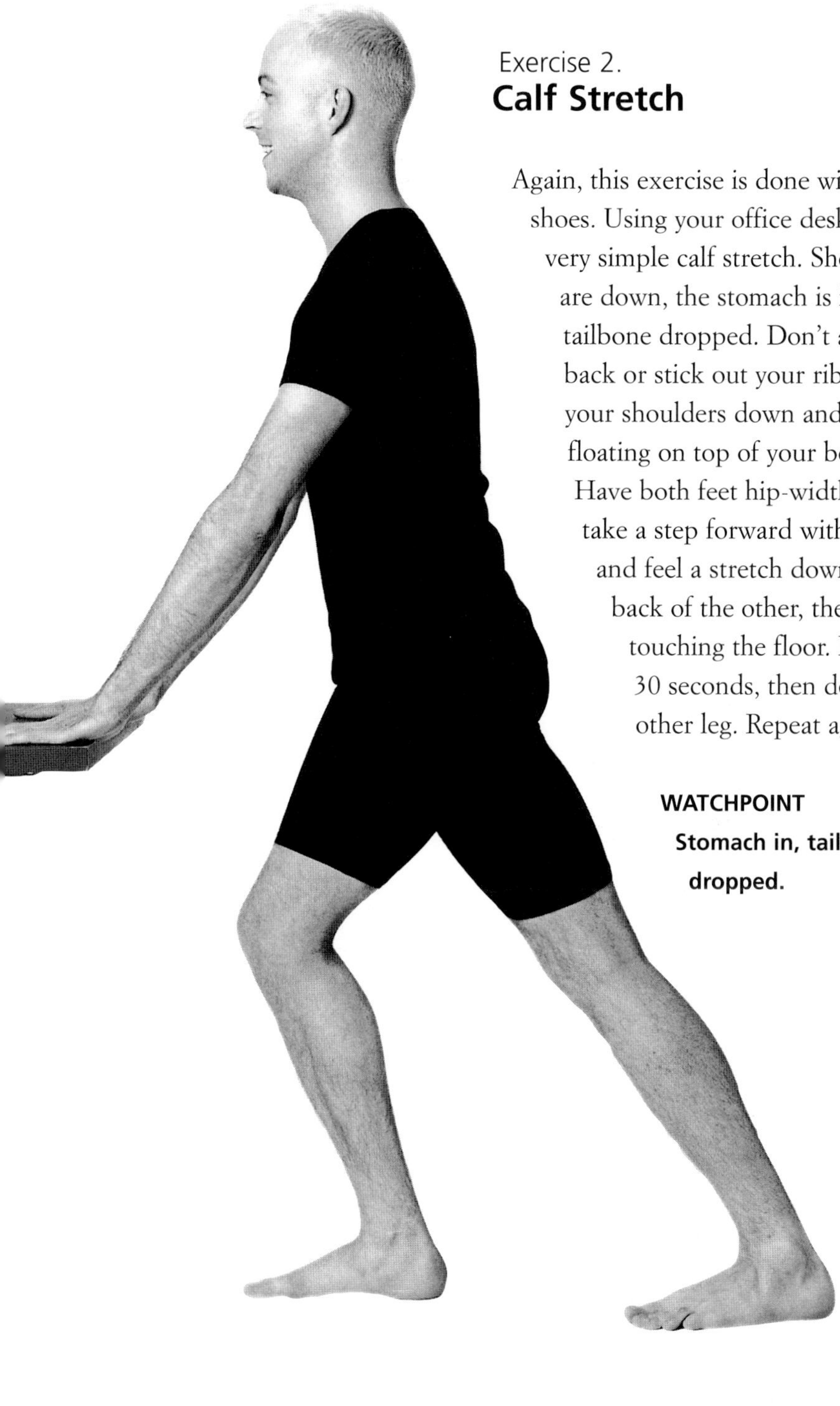

Exercise 2.

Calf Stretch

Again, this exercise is done without shoes. Using your office desk, take a very simple calf stretch. Shoulders are down, the stomach is in, the tailbone dropped. Don't arch your back or stick out your ribs. Keep your shoulders down and the head floating on top of your body. Have both feet hip-width apart, take a step forward with one leg and feel a stretch down the back of the other, the heel touching the floor. Hold for 30 seconds, then do the other leg. Repeat again.

WATCHPOINT

Stomach in, tailbone dropped.

Exercise 3.

Shoulder Rotation

This exercise will open up your shoulders. Shoulder rotations can be done seated in an office chair, but the preferred position is against a door frame or wall.

Lean with your knees bent and middle back against the wall, and slide down, keeping the knees bent. Your weight is placed evenly over the feet, which are not tense. Your middle back and the space between your shoulder blades touch the wall for support. Do not push your head back as you will feel your middle back and shoulder blades come off the wall.

WATCHPOINT

Keep your middle back and the space between the shoulder blades on the wall.

Breathing normally, gently place your hands on your shoulders. This exercise consists of four movements: circle arms forward, trying to get the elbows to touch, lift up towards the ears, circle as far back as you can without any of your middle back coming off the wall. When you have completed the movement, you then circle the other way. Back, up, around and down. Do 10 repetitions in each direction.

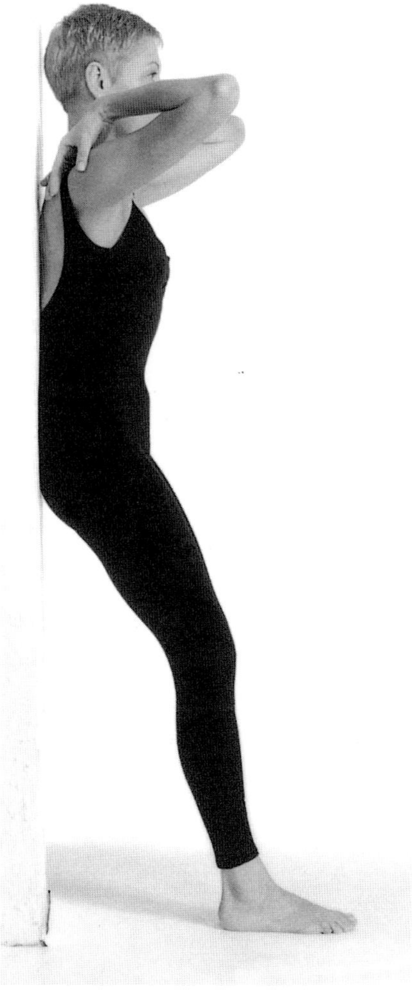

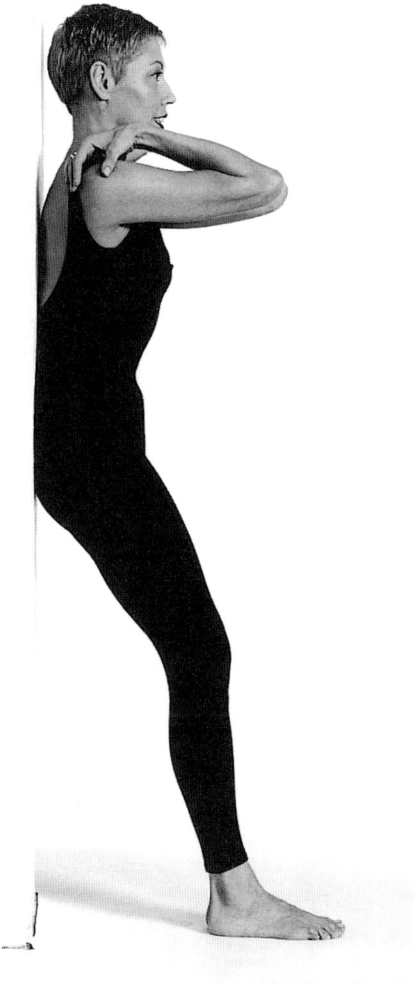

Exercises 4 & 5.

Hand Exercises

The next two exercises will help those with stiff hands or people suffering from RSI.

Sit or stand with your shoulders relaxed. Stretch your hands very gently and bring each finger to the thumb, beginning with the little finger. Stretch each of your fingers as much as you can.

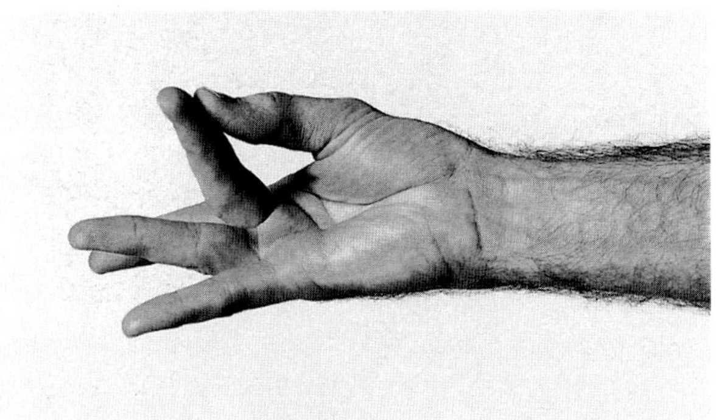

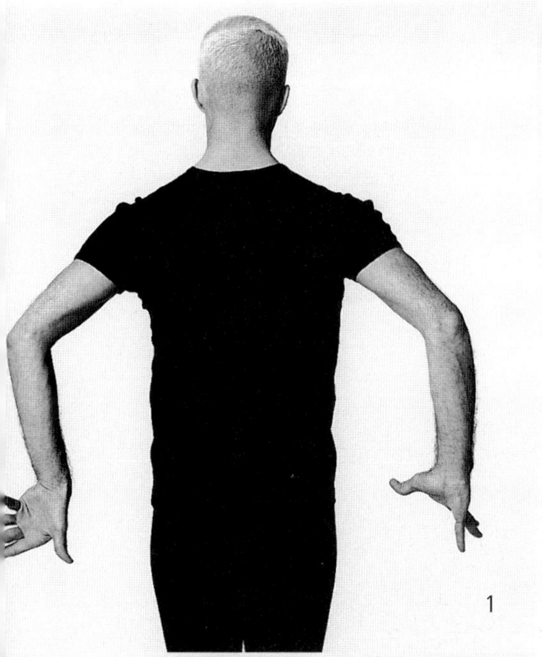

1

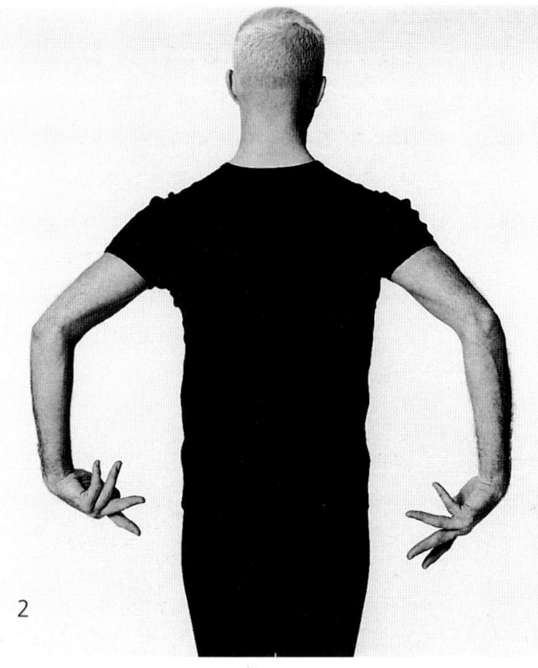

2

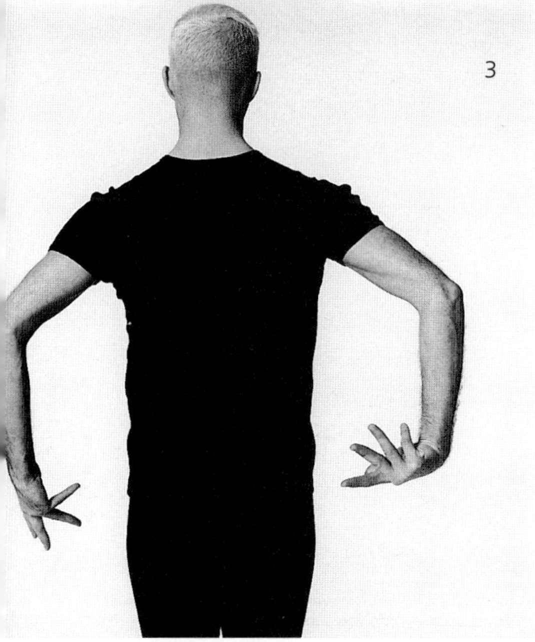

3

You can either do this exercise with your hands in front of you or behind you. The movement is exactly the same, but in this instance you circle the wrist. Think of Balinese dancers or Bob Fosse's choreography in *Chicago*. This exercise also works on coordination.

WATCHPOINT

Keep the shoulders and elbows relaxed.

Exercise 6.
Cat Stretch at the Desk

Using an office desk, this exercise will release your lower back and stretch out your shoulders. Shoes are off unless you're in flat shoes. Do not do this exercise in heels.

Stand as far away from your desk as you can while still resting your palms on the desk. Bend your knees slightly and keep them bent. Weight goes down evenly through both feet.

Breathe out, curl your chin into your chest, your stomach into your spine. Stretch out your lower back. This will counteract the effects of being seated for long periods of time, and get the blood flowing as you open your spine.

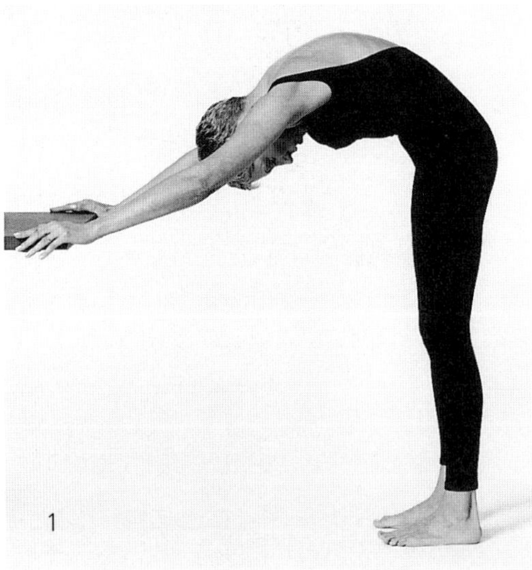

As you breathe in you press your chest down, your bottom goes up and the head gently lengthens back.

WATCHPOINT

If you feel the neck crunching or your vocal chords contracting you've taken your head too far back. There should be no discomfort in your neck.

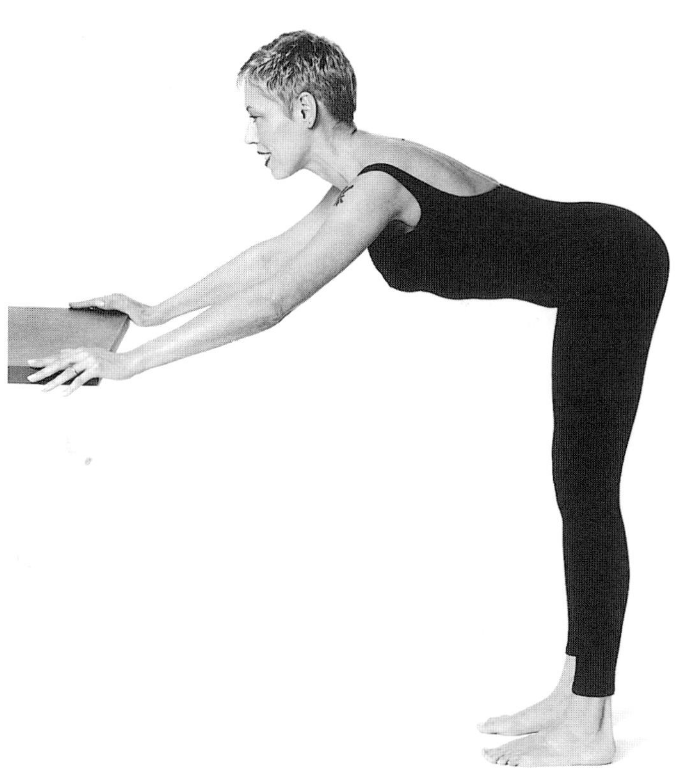

2

Exercise 7.
Shoulder Stretch

Again, stand as far away from your desk as you can with your palms resting on it. Bend your knees slightly and keep them bent. Weight goes down evenly through both feet (photograph 1).

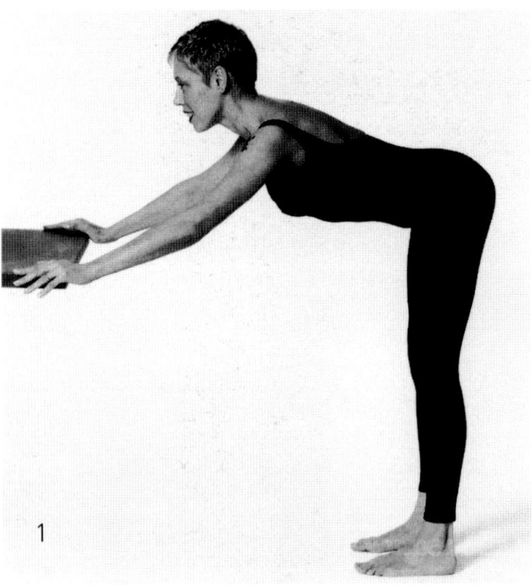
1

For this Shoulder Stretch keep the ears between the arms. Holding on to the desk, press your chest down and stretch your arms to give your shoulders, neck and upper arms a good stretch. Don't worry if you feel a little ache in your upper arms, because it is 'referred pain' from stretching out your upper back.

WATCHPOINT

Keep knees bent and head between the arms.

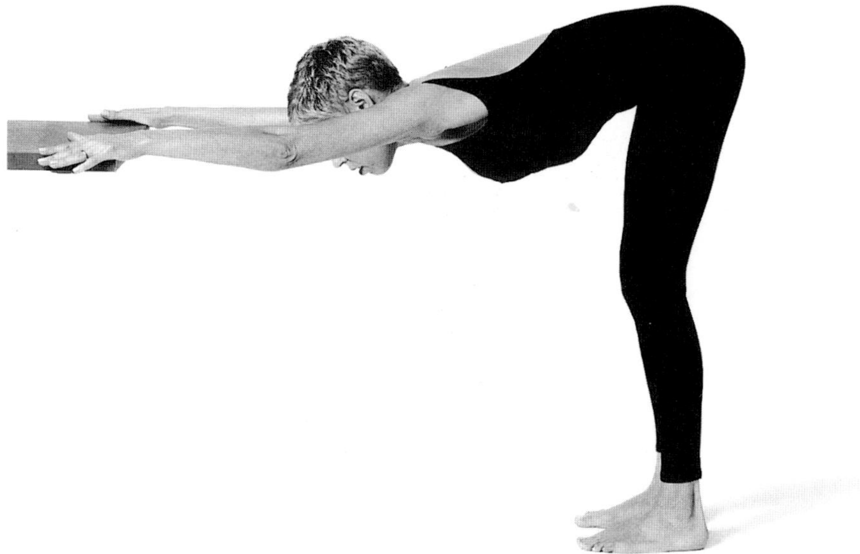

2

Pilates and martial arts

British welterweight Taekwon-do champion Jason Creighton has been taking Pilates classes for over a year. Taekwon-do, from Korea, is a stylish martial art practised by most actors in martial arts films.

'I began Taekwon-Do when I was 13. I'm semi-professional and have been competing for the past eight years. There are Taekwon-do kicks that can take someone off a horse, and jumps which bridge a 6-metre gap. It is a full contact sport, which means that you can hit someone as hard as you wish. Although punches to the face are not allowed, kicks to the head and body are.

'Frank Bruno can punch two tonnes per square inch, but that's for a sitting target. When you kick, especially with the top of the feet, you kick with the instep. It's a hard kicking surface, but it's only skin and bones underneath. If you hit someone on the point of the elbow or hip bone, something is going to break and usually it's your foot.

'An X-ray of my right foot revealed that it was broken in approximately 15 places. Many of the fractures were previous breaks that had not healed. Doctors advised me to wear an elasticized sock, and rest the foot. But I was keen to resume training.'

Fatal Mistake

'It was a fatal mistake. I'd go in and start training and the injury would not be 100 per cent healed. I'd hit it and break it again. About this time last year, I had a very bad injury in my right foot that was really preventing me from both walking and training. I went to osteopaths and physiotherapists. The podiatrist Lewis Slater looked at my feet and saw that I was standing badly. He gave me orthotic insoles and suggested I go and see Lesley. He believed Pilates would help with the injuries and begin to rebuild the muscles in my feet, so that I would start standing in the correct position and not just when I was wearing the insoles.

'My first Pilates classes were damage maintenance. As I was badly injured, I could only work with Dynabands and ankle weights. Because of Taekwon-do, I assumed that my feet and legs were my strongest physical attributes. Pilates revealed that my leg and calf muscles were compensating for weaknesses in my feet.

'Most sports concentrate on gross or large muscle movement. Pilates concentrates on fine muscle movement. There are a lot of muscles in the feet but they are very small and they make a difference to the way you stand. Lesley watched the way I was balancing and said I needed to work on the inner thigh muscles. At the time I didn't know I wasn't using the inner thigh muscles when I stood on one leg or when I kicked.'

Stable Platform

'I didn't realize that I was standing incorrectly. However, due to my Taekwon-do training I knew the theory: you must have a stable platform. If you have one side that's tense and one side that isn't, then you're riding on the outside of the leg. The fact that my foot is tilted out means that the muscles on the outside have to stay tense and these were acting more like a suspension bridge. By reversing my weight from the outside of the foot to over the second toe, I changed the way I stood. The result was increased balance and coordination. It was a process that began with gentle exercise.

'Initially my Pilates exercises were to strengthen the foot. I did a lot of Doming exercises, in which you try to lift the arch and the foot. I then moved on to coordinate the ankle and leg, flexing the ankle to a certain degree and bending the knee.

'Pilates tries to get all the muscles to work together. You use a lighter weight to perfect the coordination of a particular movement. Then, when you use the bigger weights the motion is there already. Therefore you don't have to think about the way the legs or muscles work. They work together almost automatically.

'I believe this level of coordination and balance is vital for athletes. Most people don't realize how lucky they are to be able to walk correctly. This is the difference between a person who is a fantastic sprinter and another runner who is not. Both have the same strength, but one could be standing on the wrong point of the foot so that the muscles aren't working in unison.'

Fine Tuning

'At high levels of competition everyone essentially has the same skills. They have the same strength, the same weight. They train as hard. Getting the edge depends on the fine-tuning of both movement and balance. You can never have too much balance.

'Because of the attention to detail, I found Pilates to be completely different to my other training. I do many of the same exercises over and over again, and there's a gradual progression, but sometimes that's difficult to perceive. I like vigorous and punishing exercise. Only then do I feel like I'm doing something – I'm sweating and my brain releases all those endorphins.

'Pilates is not about effort, it's about perseverance. I also noticed that on the days that I did Pilates I also trained better in Taekwon-do. I now use a Dynaband and do simple Pilates exercises before competitions. I make a point of observing an opponent's stance. You can't determine, by looking at someone's face, whether he's a good or bad fighter, but by observing the areas from the knee down to the foot, you will have a good sense of his abilities.'

Visualization

'I had been using the technique of visualization long before I came to Pilates. When I do an exercise for the first time, I try to picture myself doing it. Research was carried out on basketball players. They tied muscle sensors around their arms and documented which muscles were used for free throws. When basketball players were asked not to do a free throw, but to visualize them instead, the research showed that 70 per cent of the muscles were actually working during visualization.

'As a rule I don't tell my competitors about Pilates, although I encourage the people I train with to use the method. Most athletes, if they're really good, have to concentrate on the fine aspects of their movement. That's the ultimate in strength and movement. The skill is to place your foot in the right position, as you can then maximize the strength in your legs. A good athlete makes the motion look easy and natural as everything is working together. Pilates is helping me with that. It has made me conscious about the way I stand, and where the weight is balanced. It is making me a better martial artist.'

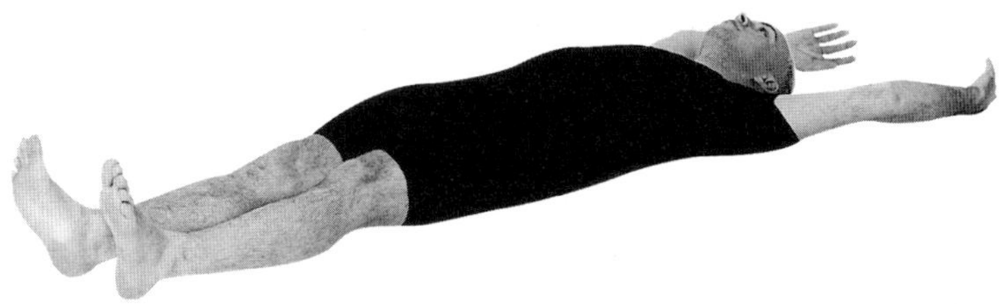

Step 4
Evening energizer

This 10- to 15-minute end-of-the-day stress release and energizer may be done before you leave your workplace or at home. You should give yourself time to 'switch off' between your working environment and your leisure time, where you transform yourself from your working mode into one of relaxation, ready to enjoy the evening.

By using breath to revive and regenerate, these exercises will energize under-used parts of the body, such as the spaces between the vertebrae. The cyclical flow of breath will reaffirm your centre, working on the coordination of the entire body, moving the body as a whole.

Compared with the previous steps, this one is more complicated. There's a pelvic tilt, with a release as well. There's a back exercise, but it's an arched back exercise. Step 4 addresses how the breath works, and the opening out of the spine. Conversely, these exercises will also address how we are inhibited in our pelvic region. Women especially may have tension in their pelvic region because of the underlining sexual aggression they encounter in public. The result is inhibition and self-consciousness on their part. Step 4 focuses on release.

WATCHPOINT

If you have a bad back, replace the Evening energizer with Step 9: Morning maintenance for bad backs.

Exercise 1.
Advanced Pelvic Tilt

This exercise will stretch out your spine and release tension in your lower and upper back, the neck, hip flexes and buttocks. It will also put you more in touch with your core and centre of gravity.

Lie on a towel or a soft surface with a small towel folded high up behind your cranium, not behind your neck. The neck is long and in neutral. Knees are comfortably bent, feet on the floor, hip-width apart, energy equally grounded through both feet, toes lengthened. There is no tension in your buttocks, the tailbone is heavy.

Breathe in and out a few times and feel your spine relaxing into the floor. Don't force your spine down or your pelvis forward or backward, allow it to settle into its natural neutral position, which is different for all of us. The arms are beside you, palms facing down.

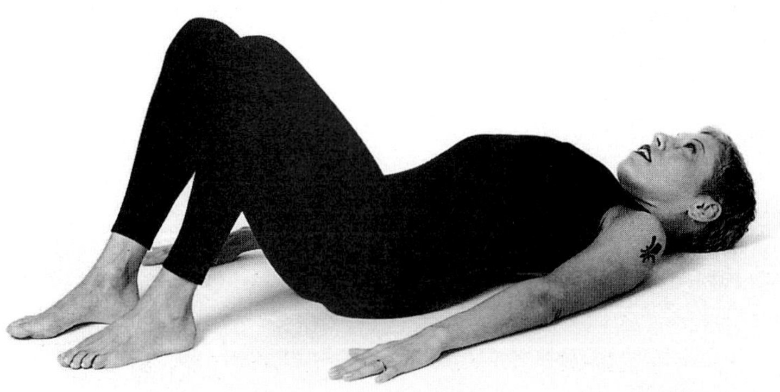

As you breathe out, very gently roll up one vertebra at a time onto your shoulders. Only go as high as the ribs are soft and the chin does not tip backward. If the ribs are lifted and the chin tips back you have gone too high for your spinal mobility, but this will improve in time.

As you breathe out, roll up one vertebra at a time, tucking the pelvis under, using the primary curve in the lumbar spine. Then, gently breathing in, bring the arms over the head. Only take the arms as far back as the neck doesn't drop backward. This depends on the mobility of your shoulders. Then very gently breathe out and roll down from the top of your spine one vertebra at a time. Think of your sternum – the breastbone – relaxing into the mat – again one vertebra at a time. You relax your chest and the base of the spine touches the floor last. Bring the arms back to their starting position.

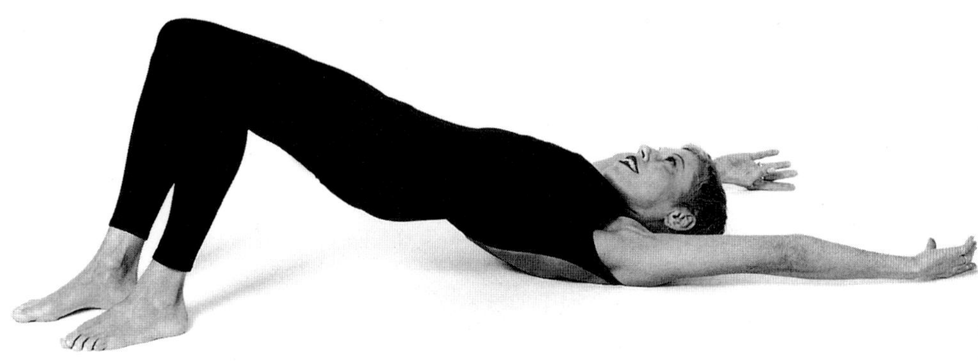

The second half of the movement is a very gentle release going the other way. Thus, gently arching, so that the lower back leaves the mat and relaxes down. Again, if your chin drops backward, you've lifted too high. The buttocks, head and shoulders stay on the mat. To begin with, you might not be able to extend a reverse arch very far.

Repeat 10 times.

WATCHPOINT

None of these exercises should be done with a bad back.

Exercise 2.

Roll-Up

Lie on your back with your feet gently flexed and legs straight, take the arms behind the head. The middle back stays on the mat the entire time so you might not be able to take your hands too far back.

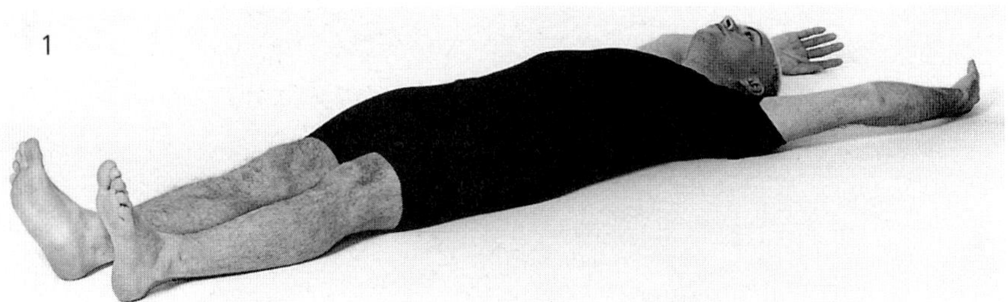
1

Very gently breathe out and bring the arms forward so they're touching the side of your thighs. Breathe in, lift your head, chin towards the chest, then breathe out and use your abdominal muscles to curl up one vertebra at a time and very gently relax and stretch over your legs to stretch out your back and hamstrings.

Breathe in and come up to a seated position, sitting tall (photograph 2). The tailbone is heavy. Gently roll down again one vertebra at a time. Do this exercise 10 times.

WATCHPOINT

Think of your energy going through the heels, not through the front of the thighs, so you're engaging your hamstrings as stabilizers.

Use your stomach as the main initiator of the movement. As you stretch forward on the final point of the exercise, the exercise becomes a lower back and hamstring stretch (photograph 3). The more you flex your feet up to your knees the more you will actually stretch out the tension in your hamstrings which has been built up from standing and sitting all day.

2

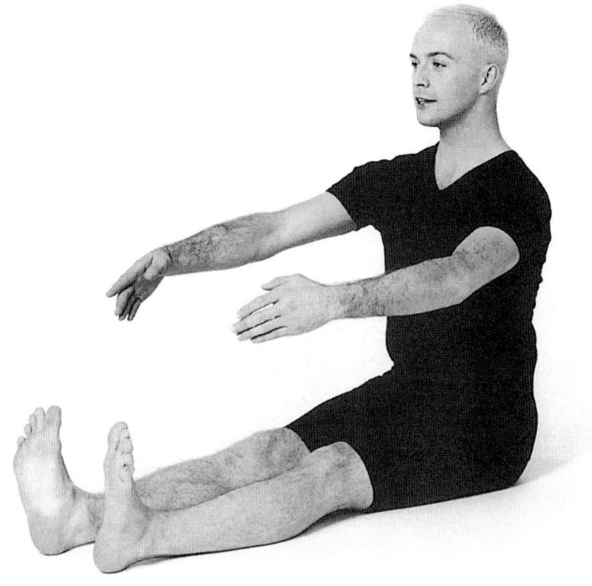

3

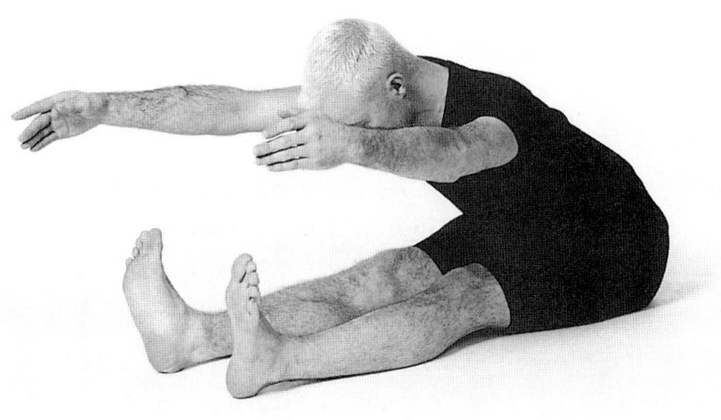

Exercise 3.
Complicated Cat Stretch

Make a square of the body with the knees hip-width apart and the hands gently resting under the shoulders.

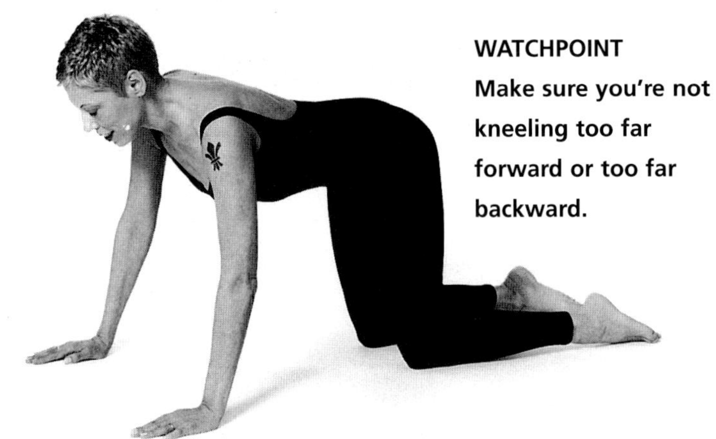

WATCHPOINT
Make sure you're not kneeling too far forward or too far backward.

1

The feet are relaxed and the hands are under the shoulders. Keep the elbows softly bent. Breathe out and pull your stomach in and curl back like a cat, tucking your chin onto your chest, bottom onto your heels. Breathe in and bend your elbows so you stretch your chest towards the floor. As you come through again, the head gently lifts, but not so far that you feel your neck crunch or the vocal chords contract.

Then reverse: stomach in, breathe out in a wave-like motion, stretch back onto the heels, curl your stomach into the spine, stretch out the lower back as you bend the elbows and release forward, pressing the chest to the floor.

Repeat 10 times.

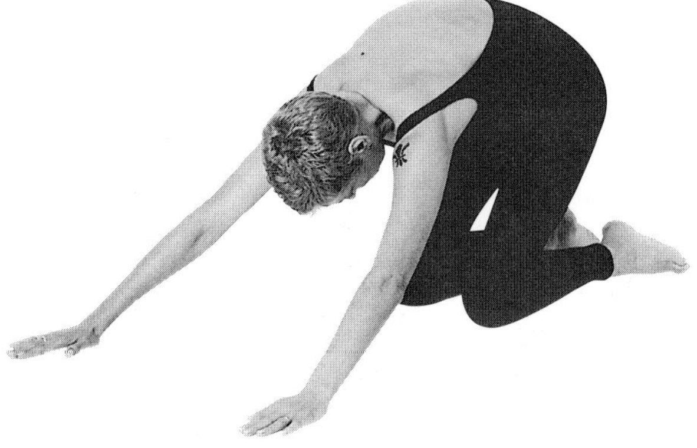

2

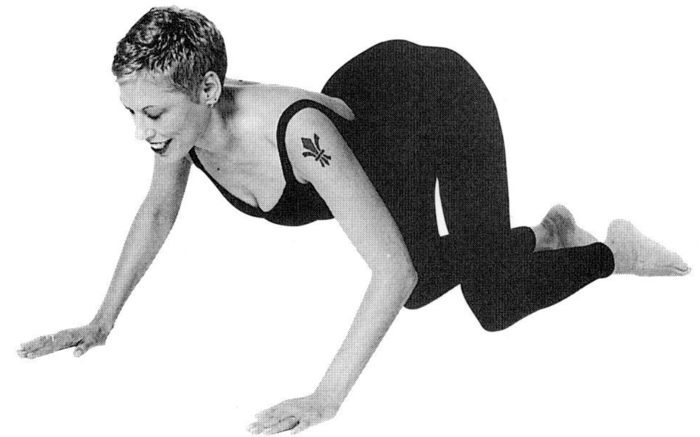

3

Exercise 4.
Standing Side Stretch

Hold a towel rail with your right hand, lift your left hand near the ear, stretch out, bend the left knee and feel a side stretch. Hold for four seconds and come back, changing sides.

Make sure your stomach is in and your ribs aren't sticking out to ensure that you are not arching your lower back. You should be able to see the outside arm in the air just in front of your ear. Don't let your arm swing behind you or your back will arch.

Repeat this five times on each side.

WATCHPOINT

Hold on to something stable, like a towel rail. Make sure that your right hand is slightly lower than your shoulder. As you breathe out, very gently let your weight move towards the top hip.

1

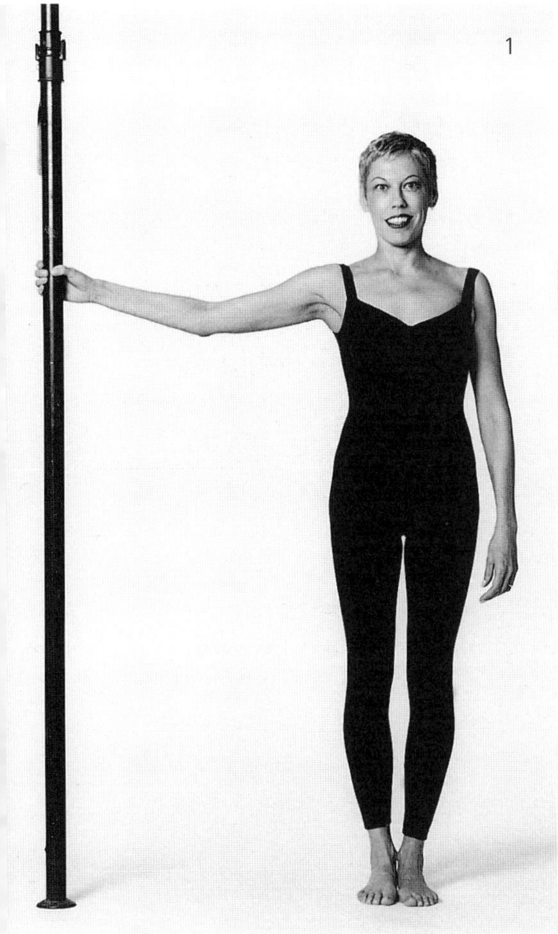

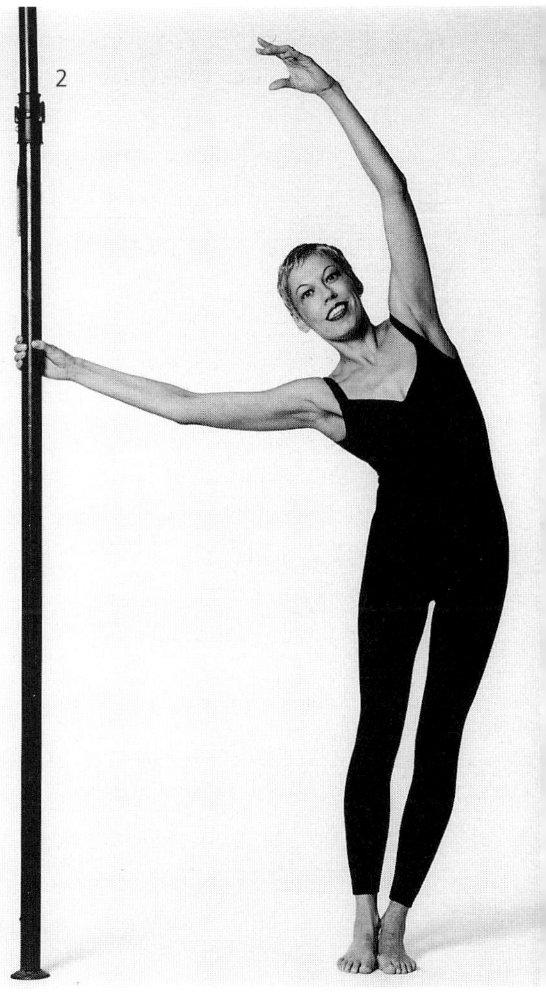

2

Writers and back pain

'Historically writers have bad backs,' explains Snoo Wilson, the playwright who takes his Pilates class at the end of his working day, which consists of sitting at a desk and writing. Pilates was recommended to him by another writer who has scoliosis. Snoo has been taking classes at Body Maintenance for the past three years.

'Writing is very much in the head. You go to Pilates and you have to concentrate on your body in an absolute way. It's a discipline that I'm not accustomed to. I don't pay attention to my body. If I had paid attention to my body in the last 50 years I wouldn't have to deal with these postural problems.'

Inherited Back Problems

'My postural problems were inherited from my father who had a bad back. I also had a fever that went into my hip a few years ago, and I think my problem started there. Something went off balance. My right side is more vulnerable than the left. I think all those things tend to give you a muscular compensation, so even if you are out of kilter, you can compensate somewhat cleverly, rather than going into spasm which is the natural body reaction.

'Initially I progressed slowly in Pilates. There wasn't a huge improvement in six months, but I saw other people getting better and I trusted the way Lesley added on exercises. She knew what was going on, and after a year there was a good improvement, which has sort of continued.

'What I've got is an ongoing problem which is manageable. Previously I was pretty stymied all the time. I'm very happy to do Pilates, and if I have to do it for the rest of my life, fine. You're coping with a disability. I envy people so much who have better mobility. But there are so many things happening in the world, that having a bad back and actually being able to deal with it should be regarded as a privilege.'

Magic Bullet

'I usually take class at 5 pm. Pilates is not a magic bullet for everything. Sometimes I feel energized and sometimes after I finish I feel tired. It does vary, as does the amount of strength you have. It differs enormously from day to day depending upon whether I've been doing something physical. It all does seem to come from a state of mind or the planets.

'When I do feel energized I attribute it to exercising. You approach your body as a united energy field. Everything that deals with the body on a holistic level like that sooner or later ends up in a quasi-contemplative ideology, which one strives towards in one's rather Westernized way. It's not like an endorphin rush. My overall well-being has improved during Pilates, which has to do with structured exercise and some different kind of bodily awareness.

'And sometimes, it's great not to be in pain.'

Pilates Master class

Before *10-Step Pilates* addresses general body toning and strengthening, Nick Ringham will here review key Pilates concepts. A former ballet dancer with Sadler's Wells, Nick started doing Pilates as an injured dancer and decided to train in the method. An associate and instructor at the Body Maintenance Studio, he has a dancer's meticulous attention to exercise detail and a personal understanding of severe back pain. He stresses the basics to his students and his innate understanding of the human body makes him an excellent teacher.

Breathing

For Nick, the beginning is always breath:

'There is a saying that comes from Yoga, which is "if there is no breath there is no life". I think that says a lot.

'You must breathe regularly when you exercise because you must oxygenate your body. You must get oxygen into the muscles so that you can replenish energy, and as a result, create the power to enhance strength and flexibility. Aside from a purely physical level, breathing used during Pilates can be inspiring, mood-altering, and sometimes even life-changing. Quite often we have physical and emotional things locked up in our bodies that we're not even aware of, and breathing and exercise can have an almost therapeutic effect.'

Nick believes that breathing is intricately connected to emotional states:

'If one was to sit down – without doing Pilates – and concentrate only on breathing, it has the meditative effect of cutting off the internal dialogue going on in your head. Just by controlling your breathing you can create an emotional state. If you employ a very shallow or rapid breath, you can become nervous or irritable. With Pilates, we try to slow the breath down, to relax and focus, thus releasing tension from our bodies. People don't associate tranquillity with physical exercise. Following a Pilates session your muscles may feel a little worked, tight here and stretched there, but you leave with an overall feeling of well-being.'

Increased Coordination

Another real benefit of Pilates is increased coordination.

'The technical term is "proprioceptive", which is your brain's connection with your body. Let's suppose that you are walking along and you trip up on an uneven pavement. If the connections between your mind and body are reasonably good and your coordination is fair you are going to recover that step rather quickly, without even thinking about it.

'It's surprising how disconnected we are, and people who aren't proprioceptively aware and have poor musculature will miss that step and possibly fall.'

Sadler's Wells

Nick trained in classical ballet as a youth. His first injury took place after he was called in to replace another injured ballet dancer during an end-of-year ballet school performance, doing the other dancer's work as well as his own. All he remembers was that the pain was so acute he had to ask for the car to be stopped on the way home and get out. Afterwards he rested for six weeks and was fine, or so he thought.

By the time he was 18 he was dancing for Sadler's Wells and didn't have any problems for the next four years. A relapse occurred after a long tour. During a cossack dance with split jumps and back jumps in Stravinsky's ballet *Petrouchka*, Nick's back seized up as he jumped into the air and bent backwards. Unable to land properly, he jarred the whole of his spine.

He was only able to leave hospital after a doctor put a shot of novocaine into his spine. Afterwards he tried acupuncture, which eliminated some pain, but only for a short while. Nick continued dancing for several more years, but always with back pain.

Even though Nick knew about Pilates from other dancers, he always felt that dance training by itself should have been enough to strengthen his body, if he worked hard enough. When he started to take Pilates classes with Alan Herdman, Nick was in for a surprise. Classical ballet requires extreme external rotation in the hip socket, and for many people, this is not possible. Dancers often cheat and therefore end up with problems in the lower back, as well as difficulties with knees, ankles and feet due to forced turnout.

'Through Pilates, I discovered how my body was imbalanced from one side to the other. For example, one hip turned out and the other hip didn't. One side of my body was stronger but tighter, and the other side of my body was more supple but weaker.'

Perseverance

Even for a dancer like Nick, doing Pilates was frustrating in the beginning.

'Sometimes while attempting to do abdominal work, my back became painful and I had to be careful. I didn't want to push it to the point of aggravating the back problem while trying to strengthen the abdominals. On some days my back would be quite loose and I could work reasonably hard, on others my back would start tweaking and hurting a bit. I'd think, "Am I doing this wrong? Or maybe I shouldn't be doing this."'

From his own experience, Nick realized the importance of persevering and finding new ways of working.

'I'm not suggesting that people should find a different exercise. I mean alternating the same exercise to suit the problem. So you don't tense up your back area while doing a low-impact abdominal exercise, which is entirely possible. Sometimes it takes quite a lot of relearning in order to do something as simple as that.'

Visualization

Nick also believes strongly in the power of visualization.

'I definitely do it myself. I quite often use the idea of breathing or filling or emptying the body with breath, a bit like the waves of the sea coming in, filling up and rushing back out again. That visualization is very relaxing whether you are lying down relaxing or whether you are doing a stretch. Sometimes when I relate this to my students they think, "What is he talking about?" But I do think visualization is important because it takes the exercising and breathing on to another plane rather than just the physical.'

Patience and Pilates

'When learning to do these exercises one might reach a point of understanding what you're aiming for, but while doing it, it might still be frustrating because your body is not doing what you're telling it to do. Don't give up, even though it seems very difficult. There will come a time when it will change. Pilates requires patience.'

With his own back injury Nick felt some changes immediately, which made him keep going back to Pilates.

'But for a big, big change I had stopped dancing and was working intensely in Pilates for a good year. Then I really noticed a change in my body shape, the feel, the way I was holding myself and the way I related to my centre.'

Teaching for a Decade

For the past 10 years Nick has been teaching Pilates.

'Once I decided to stop dancing I was left with quite a void, as many former dancers will tell you. Because suddenly you realize that ballet has been all-encompassing for your image, your life and your world. Take that away, it can be a little scary.'

Pilates continues Nick's ongoing work with the body, except the body in question is not just his own.

'Initially I started to teach from a dancer's point of view, but I soon realized that not everybody comes from that background, and therefore their physical problems would be different. Over the years my teaching ability has grown and I can now work with people from all walks of life, just as we do at the Body Maintenance Studio.'

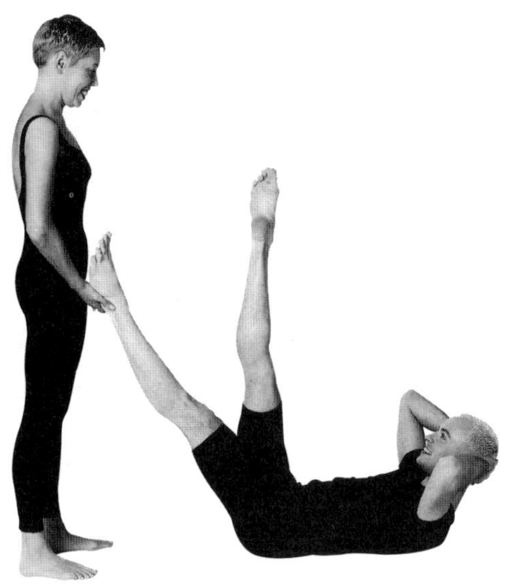

Step 5
Tummy toner

This second half of the book will focus on toning and strengthening.

Women are often obsessed with having flat stomachs like men, regardless of the obvious physical differences. These exercises, combined with careful and healthy eating, will tone and tighten the stomach area. They will not make you lose weight, but they will give you a flatter, leaner stomach.

As people age, their metabolism changes and they must exercise more to burn up the same amount of calories. By exercise, I mean walking instead of taking the car or a bus, or climbing the stairs instead of taking a lift. If you're short-waisted and eat large meals, you are going to have a stomach that protrudes. It is better for your blood sugar levels to eat small amounts throughout the day. Also allow yourself some flexibility, and don't obsessively deny yourself certain foods.

However, the more fats and sugars you ingest, the more you need to exercise to maintain your target weight. Visualize the way you wish to be. If you imagine yourself to be lean and energized, you need a lifestyle that complements that image. There are certain ways of eating and amounts of exercise that will make you feel more positive. Try to become aware of a diet and lifestyle which suit your body, and adjust yourself accordingly. What's required is to change what you eat to achieve your body's natural, healthy balance.

In Pilates when you do your abdominal work, as you breathe in the stomach gently expands. As you breathe out the stomach pulls in, navel to spine. Feel the connection from the pubic bone up to the navel. The body will automatically want to do the opposite as you breathe out on the point of effort. You inhale through the nose and exhale through the mouth. As you breathe out you think about pulling the navel to the spine without tipping the pelvis. If you have trouble with the pelvis and you have tight hip flexes and glutes, go to the section of the leg stretches where you stretch your bottom with the foot on the thigh, and do one or two of those stretches first to relax your pelvis (see pages 120 and 121).

A strong stomach exists to support your internal organs and back. The taller you stand, the more balanced your stance, the flatter your stomach will appear. When you are posturally aligned and maintaining an erect back while walking, you are exercising your body perfectly well. If you sit slouched all the time and if you walk with a slump, your stomach will stick out.

Exercise 1.
Basic Sit-Up

Lie on your back with your legs comfortably against a wall or with your feet held up by a friend, legs gently rotated in the hip sockets. Be close enough to, or far away enough from the wall so that your tailbone is weighted to the mat. If your bottom is off the ground you're too close to the wall. Conversely, if you're too far away your legs won't feel supported.

1

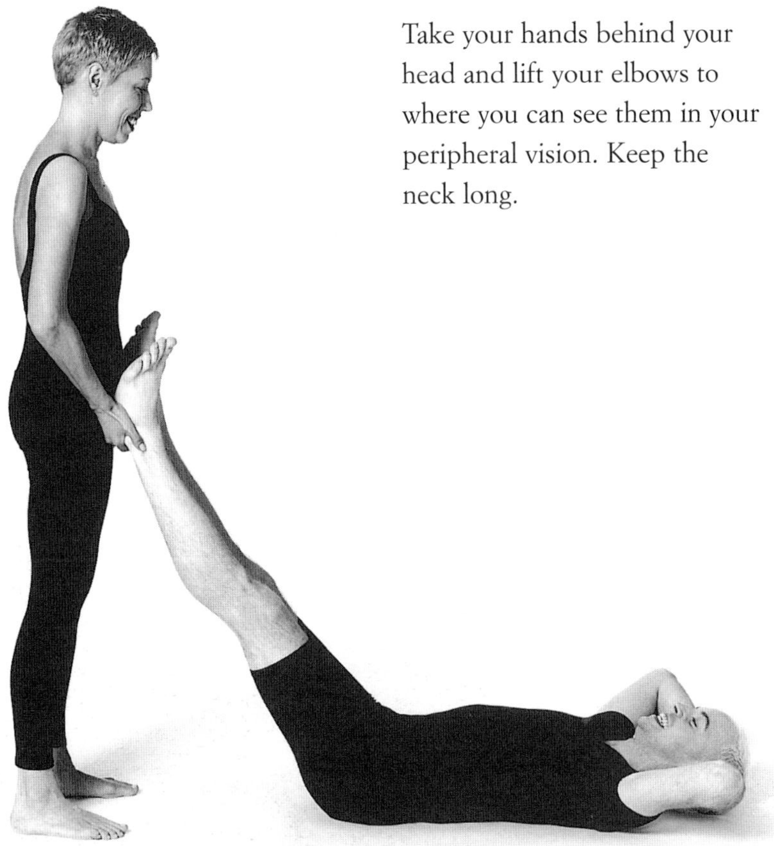

Take your hands behind your head and lift your elbows to where you can see them in your peripheral vision. Keep the neck long.

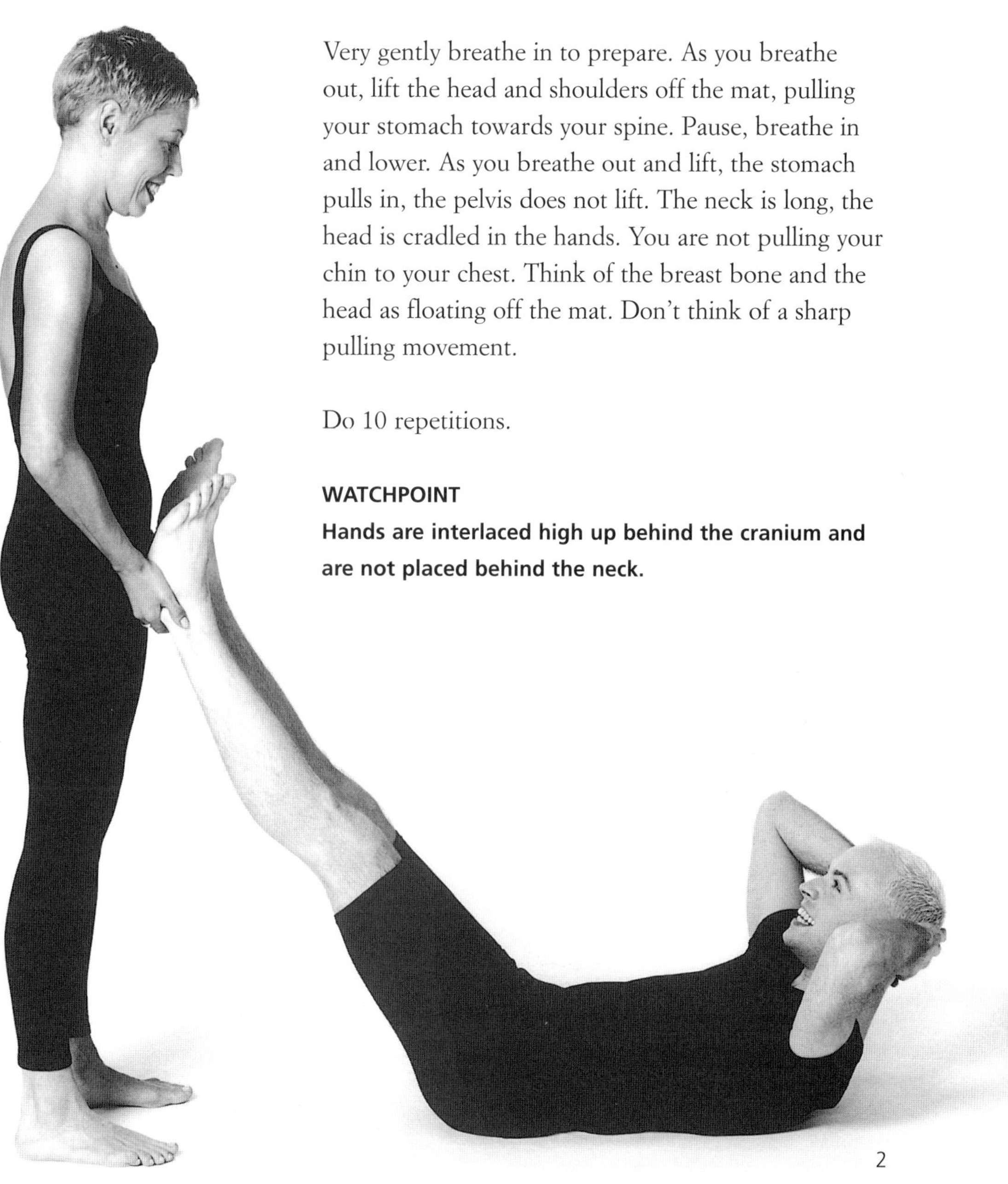

Very gently breathe in to prepare. As you breathe out, lift the head and shoulders off the mat, pulling your stomach towards your spine. Pause, breathe in and lower. As you breathe out and lift, the stomach pulls in, the pelvis does not lift. The neck is long, the head is cradled in the hands. You are not pulling your chin to your chest. Think of the breast bone and the head as floating off the mat. Don't think of a sharp pulling movement.

Do 10 repetitions.

WATCHPOINT

Hands are interlaced high up behind the cranium and are not placed behind the neck.

2

Exercise 2.
Basic Sit-Up with Leg Lift

Assume the same position as in the previous exercise.

Breathe out, and lift off the mat. Pause, breathe in. Breathe out and lift one leg away from the wall and place it back. Breathe in, breathe out, lift the other leg away from the wall and place it back. These are alternative leg lifts. Either do 10 alternating on each side without placing the head down or, if you feel a strain in the neck, do four then rest. Do another four, then rest again.

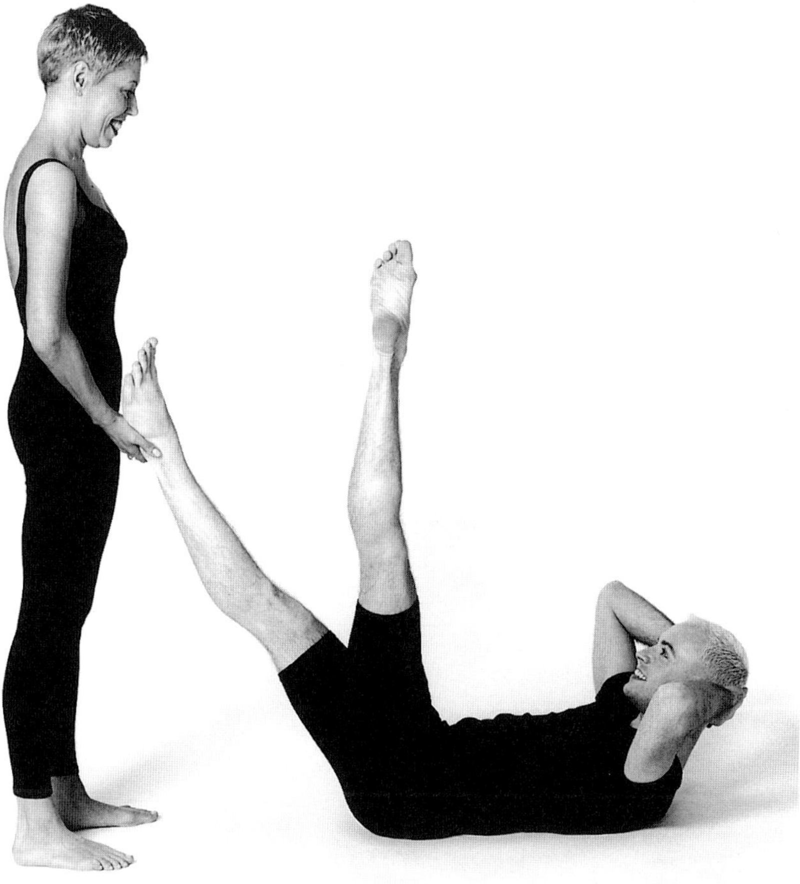

Exercise 3.

Tummy Toner with Dynaband (1)

The following exercises are done with a Dynaband, a long piece of elasticized rubber used by physiotherapists. Dynabands can be obtained through most health and fitness stores. Unlike weights, they can be easily packed for travel.

WATCHPOINT

Make sure you tie the Dynaband to something secure, such as banisters or a door knob, with the door firmly locked.

This exercise works on the stomach as well as gently working on the inside thigh.

In all of these exercises you can have a towel behind your head. The same rules apply: Lie on your back with a towel behind your head, have both knees bent. Your pelvis is heavy, there is no tipping. The back is in neutral. You are not pressing your back down, nor are you letting it arch. The arms are resting softly beside you. Think of energy reaching out through the tips of your middle finger, to relax your shoulders and lengthen your neck. Your chin is dropped forward very softly towards the throat – not tucked in. If you find this position uncomfortable you will need a towel behind the head. Your feet are relaxed.

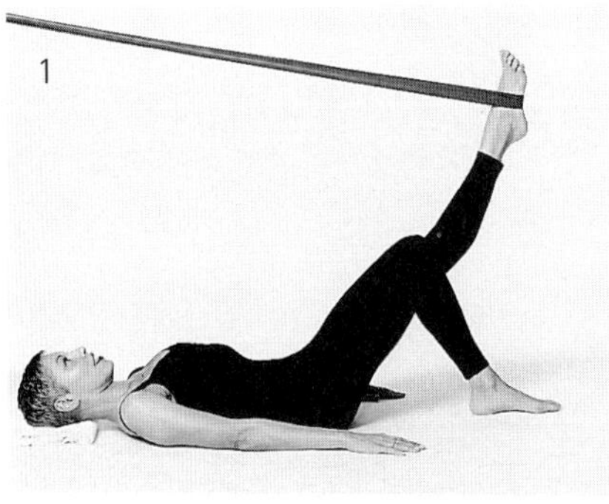
1

Place your right heel in the Dynaband. Start with your right leg straight and level with your left knee. As you breathe out, the leg lowers gently to about 6 to 8 inches (15 to 20 cm) off the ground. Breathe in and lift the leg so that it is level with the other knee.

2

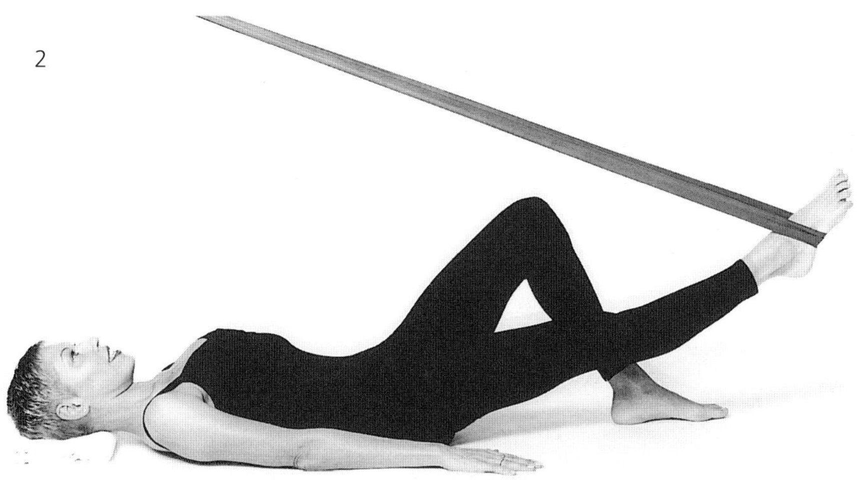

Do 10 repetitions with each leg.

WATCHPOINT

Don't take the leg too low, or you will feel your back arching or your neck shorten. Don't let the leg lift higher than the supporting knee or your pelvis will not be balanced.

A second way of doing these exercises is with your leg turned out or slightly externally rotated at the hip socket. As you turn out the working leg you keep the pelvis stable, the other leg is in parallel and you don't allow it to twist you towards the side.

As you do these exercises with your foot in the Dynaband think of your energy running through the heels and the backs of your legs. Try not to grip or use the front of your thigh. You must engage your stomach effectively in these exercises.

Exercise 4.
Tummy Toner with Dynaband (2)

If the front of your thighs are overly developed, they may be too heavy to do this exercise. This exercise is exactly the same as the previous one, but with both legs in the Dynaband.

Breathe out and lower the legs. Don't take them too low, only lift them as high as your starting position and be sure that your pelvis doesn't leave the mat. Very gently lower the legs, put your hands on your hips. As soon as the hips start to tip you've gone too low. Your back should be supported by your abdomen.

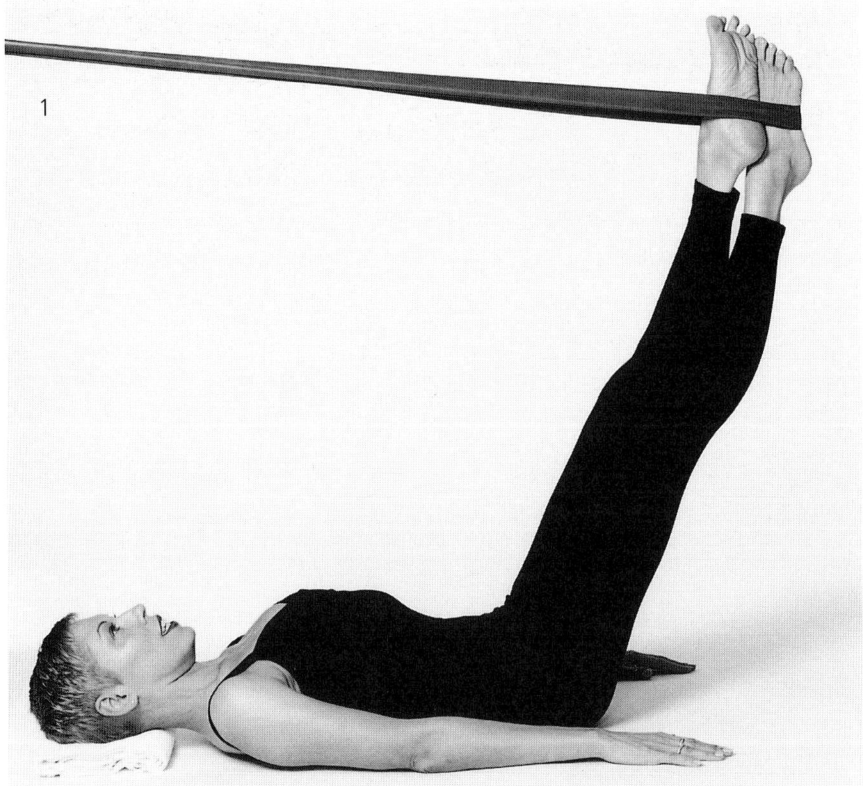

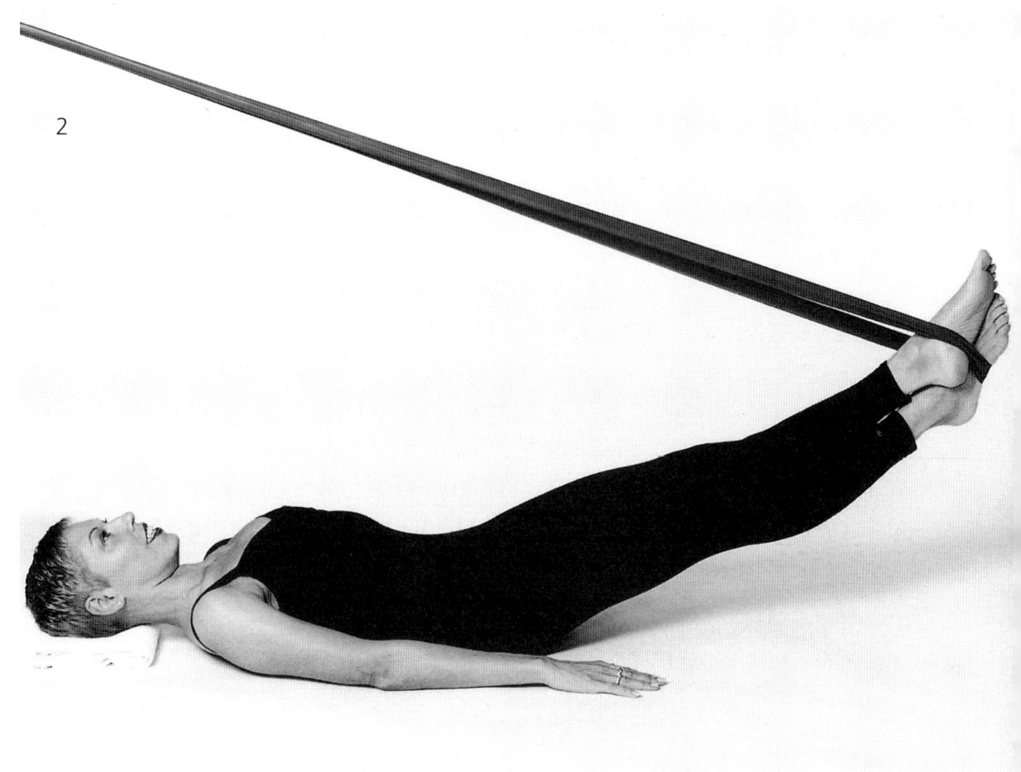

Do 10 repetitions.

Exercise 5.

Tummy Toner with Dynaband (3)

This exercise will work the inside thigh as well as the stomach. Both legs are turned out or externally rotated in the hip sockets. The right leg is on the floor turned out. Begin with the left leg in the air.

Very gently breathe out and lower the leg so the ankles almost cross. Breathe in and lift, breathe out and lower again.

Do 10 repetitions on each side.

WATCHPOINT

Make sure you don't lower the leg too low, which will cause your back to arch.

If you want to make any of these exercises more difficult, you can do them with the head lifted. The hands are interlaced and placed behind the head. Breathe in to prepare, lift the elbows to peripheral vision and breathe out as you lower the leg in any of the above exercises.

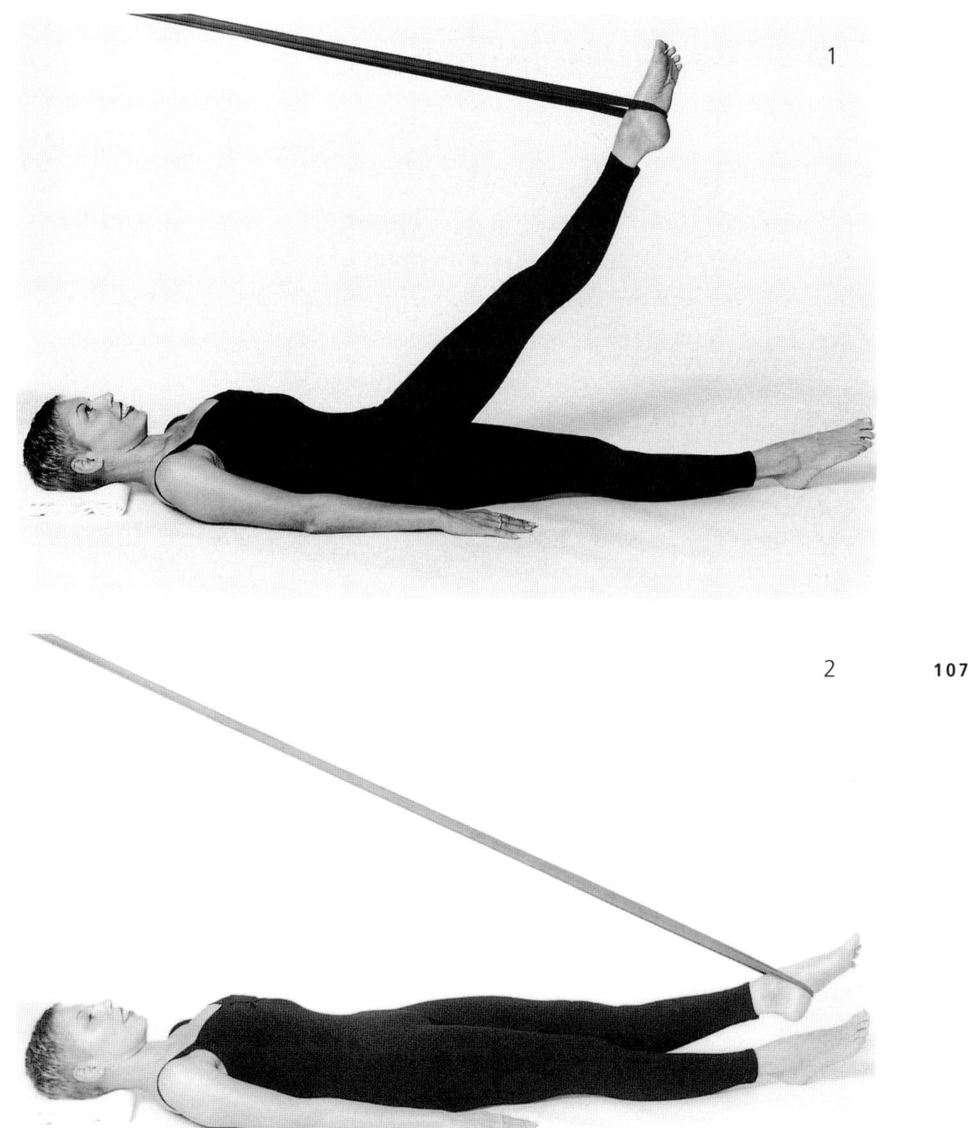
1
2

Exercise 6.
Side Stretch with Dynaband

Lie on your side in a straight line, your underneath arm flat along the floor with your ear on your arm. You might want to slide a towel between the ear and arm. The palm is flat on the ground or supporting the head (see photograph 1). The other hand is comfortably placed in front of you. Make sure you're in a straight line. Carefully bring your legs slightly further forward and you will feel your back relax. If you feel this going into your back you probably have to take the legs further forward. The hips are stacked on top of each other. It is really important not to tip either forward or backward.

Place the top foot in the Dynaband and stretch both legs quite strongly with flexed feet, the toes pointing towards the knees. The bottom foot and ankle will probably just leave the floor but your calf will stay on the floor. Very gently lift the top leg 6 to 8 inches (15 to 20 cm).

Breathe out and lower so that it touches the bottom leg.

Breathe in and lift. The effort is on the exhale as you lower the leg to touch the bottom leg. You're focusing on your stomach and waist muscles. You are also lengthening the front and back of your thigh. Again, think of the energy running through the back of the legs, not the front of the thighs. Do 10 repetitions on each side.

WATCHPOINT

Don't lock your knees.

Try to relax the top shoulder as much as possible. One of the most important things to remember about this exercise is that both legs remain the same length throughout. If one leg lengthens more than the other you will create an imbalance in the pelvis.

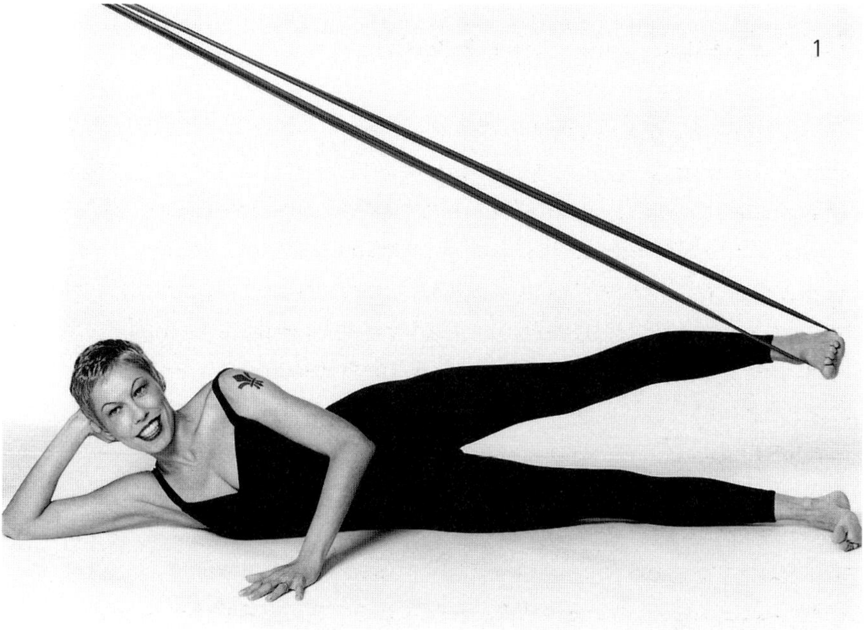

1

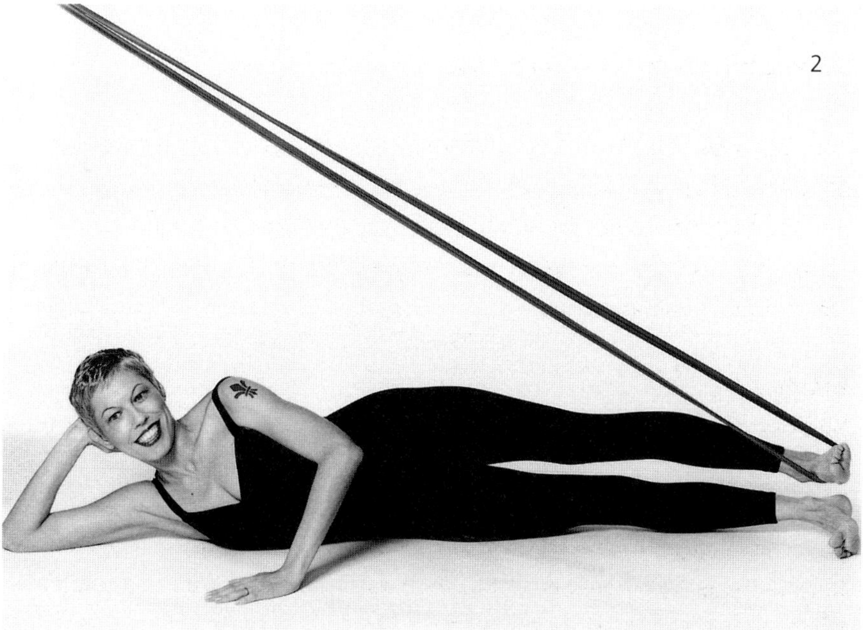

2

Pilates at the gym

Karen Cooksley runs from meeting to meeting, carrying tons of documents and briefs in her bag. A lawyer, Karen is a 10-year veteran of Pilates. She joined the Body Maintenance Studio a year after it opened. She didn't know what Pilates was, but she found it to be immediately beneficial.

'At that time I had done sports in school, but I hadn't really done any exercise during university. When I was 24, I decided I wanted to get into shape again. I used to go to the Pineapple studio for classes. Lesley Ackland had been an instructor who did general floor exercises classes. Obviously she was developing her interest in Pilates. When I was told she was running the Body Maintenance Studio I went up there, had a look, and started lessons. My tone rapidly improved and, more importantly, I found it to be a great de-stresser. As a lawyer, doing something like Pilates, which is a calm sort of exercise, is brilliant for me.'

The Stomach

'I was always very conscious of my stomach. I'm kind of curvy and quite sporty and I have a tendency to eat, drink and have a jolly time as well. So I concentrated on my stomach and tried to flatten it. A combination of running for 30 minutes and Pilates does the job. It really tucks my stomach in and makes me feel taut. When I've had an hour and a half at the Body Maintenance studio I really feel that I'm leaner and taller.

'One exercise I do after running at the gym is on my back, with my knees raised. Very slowly I bring my head and shoulders up. I breathe in and feel as if I'm wearing very tight jeans, which I zip up right to my chin. I also do sit-ups, very slowly, in a very controlled way – not those horrible crunches that make you go purple in the face, the kind you see people do in the gym.

'Pilates has made me conscious of breathing properly and stretching. I'm very conscious of not having stretched for a few days, as I feel tightness in my hips when sitting, which I would not have even noticed several years ago.'

The Obliques

'When I am in the Body Maintenance Studio I do a combination of abdominal exercises using Dynabands, and work on both the "barrel" and slope. You work your side muscles – the obliques – to pull in, across and down, which makes quite a difference to the waist. Pilates gives me that nice, waisted look.

'It also takes my mind off my work. While doing these exercises you have to think about what you're doing, concentrating on very specific parts of your body. You have to touch the button in your mind to really make it happen. So I find that I can't think about what I'm doing at work when I'm in the Body Maintenance Studio. It's a calming atmosphere. To concentrate on how to breathe properly is, in itself, very relaxing.

'That warm feeling you have inside when you walk out is different from being heated up after the gym or from doing aerobics.'

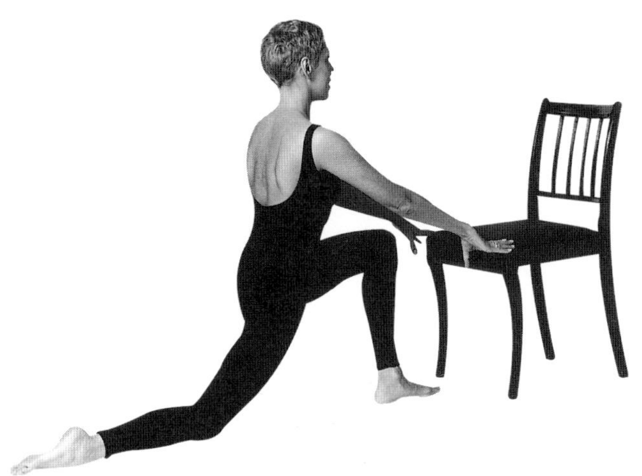

Step 6

Thigh and buttock trimmer

It is possible for people while exercising their legs to create bulk, as they do not do enough stretching. Everyone wants their leg muscles to be long, lean and lengthened as opposed to tight and bunched. There are certain parts of the legs, particularly the quadriceps muscles above the knees, that get bigger due to excessive use, while the inside thighs and the hamstrings are usually undertoned. These exercises address these problems.

The following exercises use breath not only to focus on strengthening and toning, but to lengthen the muscles as well, so that over-developed muscles become leaner and longer and under-developed ones become strong and firmer.

Exercise 1.

Inside Thigh Exercise

All the same rules apply: lie on your side, ear on the arm, the underneath palm facing the ground, the other hand in front of you gently supporting the body, the shoulders relaxed. The hips are stacked one on top of the other. You can slide a towel between your ear and your arm.

This exercise may be done with a dining room chair, using one-kilo ankle weights.

Very gently with both feet flexed, your toes pulled up towards the knees, put your top leg on the front corner of the chair. The bottom leg goes underneath the chair and slightly to the back.

As you breathe out, very gently lift the bottom leg and hold for a count of three – one, two, three. Breathe in and lower.

Do 10 repetitions on each side.

WATCHPOINT

Gently pull up the knee and stretch through the heel but don't lock the knee.

This exercise is facilitated through the stomach and the obliques, the muscles in the waist. The stomach and the obliques take the initial lift, and you then must use the inside thigh to lift the bottom leg.

1

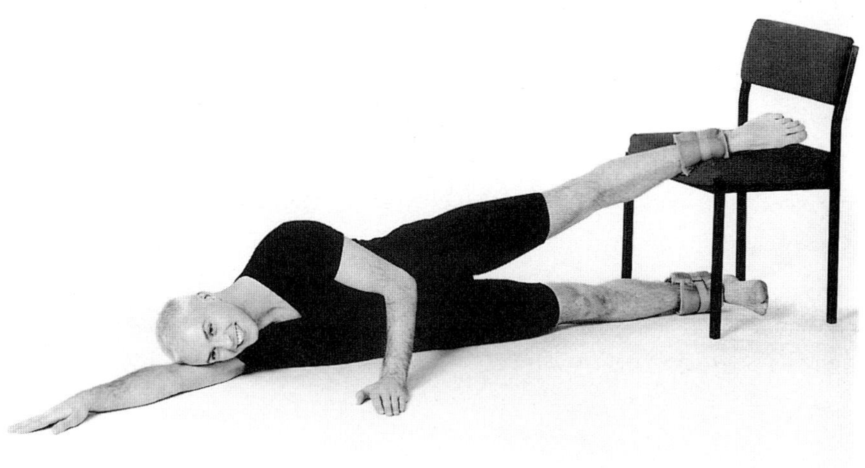

2

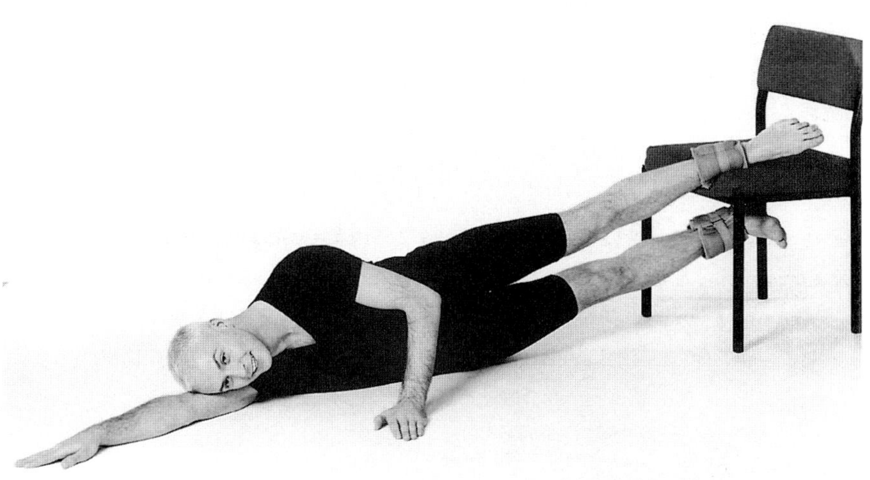

Thigh and buttock trimmer

Exercise 2.

Standing Hamstring Strengthening Exercise

This exercise will tone the backs of your legs. It can be done standing on the bottom step of a staircase, on an aerobic step or on two telephone directories piled one on top of the other.

Hold on to something solid – perhaps the wall in front of you. Think of the postural rules about standing. Hold on to the wall with your shoulders and neck relaxed. Pull the stomach in and, with the heels on the edge of the step, drop the right leg behind you. When you drop the leg don't lengthen it. Gently contract your buttock muscles together. The thighs touch and remain touching.

1

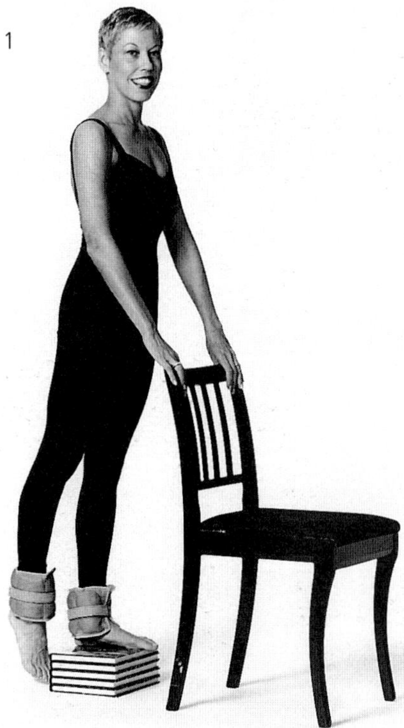

Breathe in, bend your knee as if you're going to touch your heel to your bottom, flex your foot and slowly straighten for a count of three – one, two, three – and then the toes drop below the step.

Repeat 10 times on one leg and then change legs.

WATCHPOINT

Knees remain touching, stomach stays in. As you do the exercise, make sure that you don't lean forward.

2

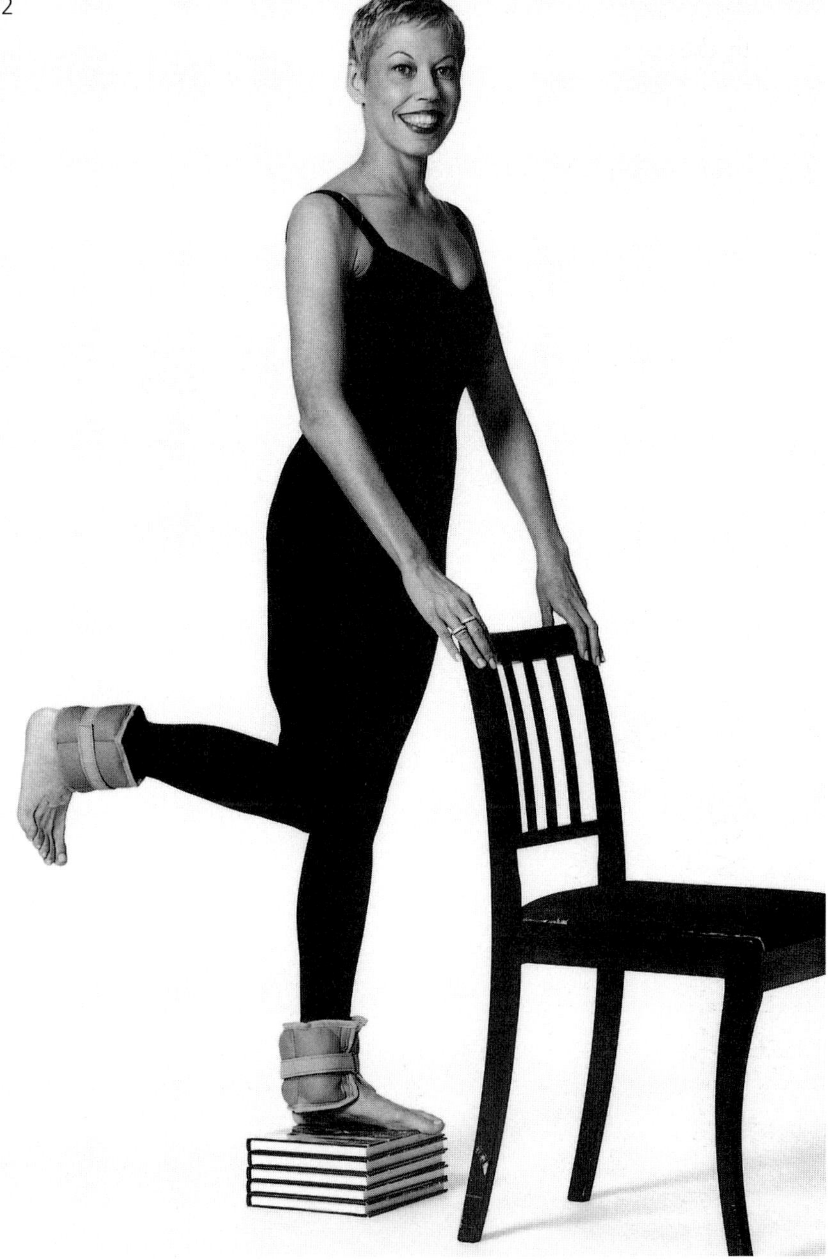

Exercise 3.
Buttock Toning Exercise

This buttock exercise will tone the under-the-cheek of your bottom. Stand in exactly the same position as the previous exercise. Squeeze the buttocks together, again without leaning forward. Gently squeeze your bottom and drop one leg behind you. Breathe out, push the leg back, breathe in and come back to centre. As you breathe out, pull your stomach in so your back doesn't arch. The foot of the working leg is flexed throughout the exercise.

10 repetitions on one leg and then change legs.

WATCHPOINT

Keep the neck long, stomach in, don't lean.

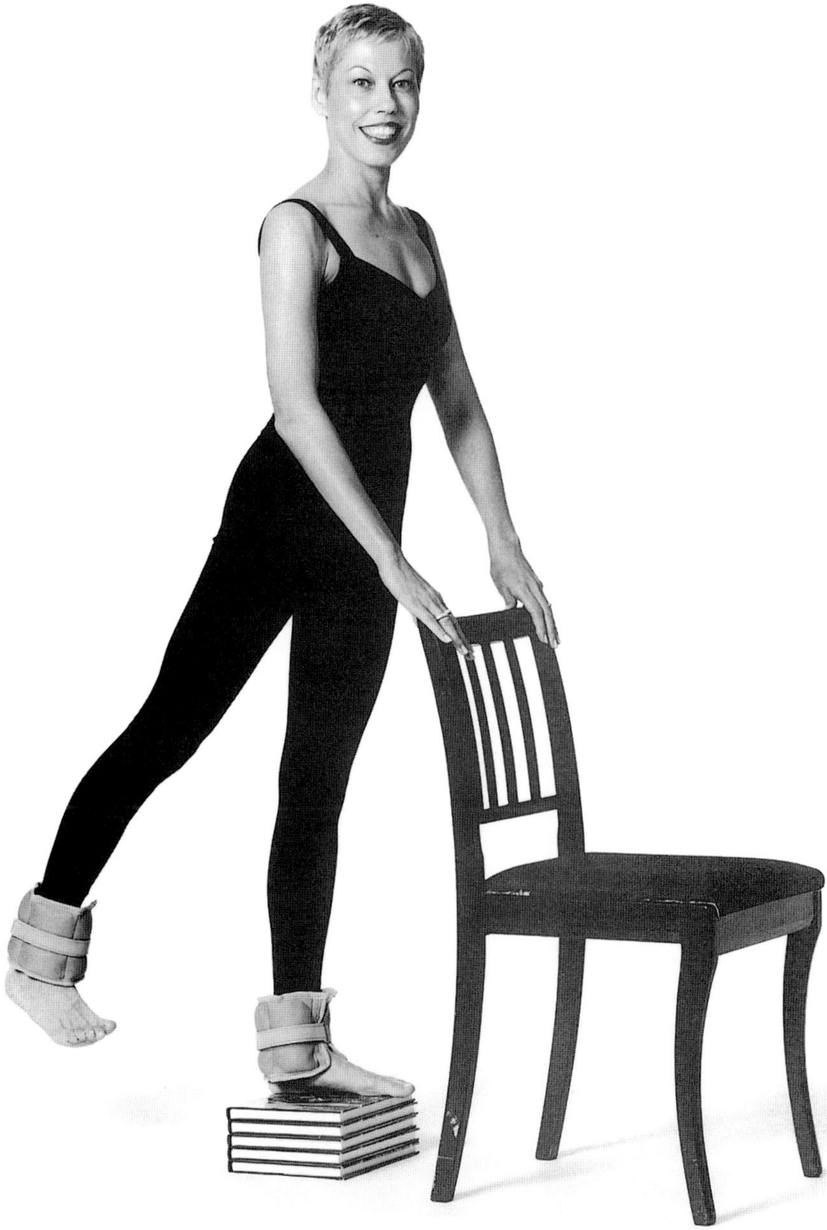

Thigh and buttock trimmer

Stretches

After the thigh and buttock exercises you need to stretch your legs. The following four stretches can be used as part of Step 1: Morning Energizer. They can also be incorporated into Step 9: Morning Maintenance for Bad Backs. These stretches may be used in any of the sections to help streamline your body. They re-create the posture, enabling the pelvis to sit naturally which can remove tightness in the buttocks, hip flexes, thighs and hamstrings. Most of us are tight because we don't do enough stretching.

All stretches are held for a minimum of 30 seconds.

Exercise 4.

Seated stretch for back of the hips and buttock exercise

Sit on a chair with both feet on the ground and cross your ankle over your knee.

1

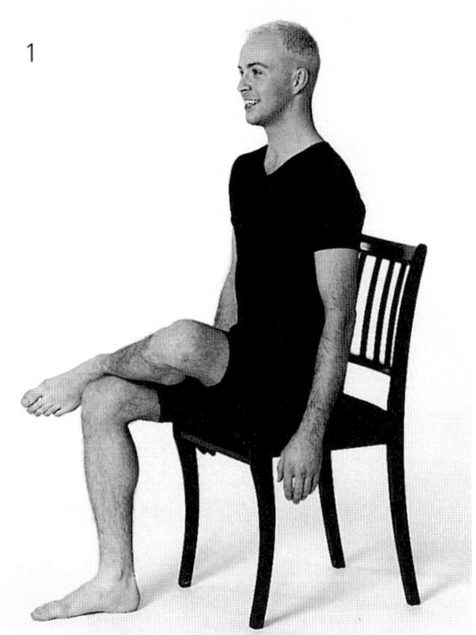

Very gently breathe out and lean forward. Try to lean over the bent knee and you will feel a stretch in the back of your hip and buttock. The head, neck and shoulders are relaxed. Gently press the raised knee down, without either pulling on your ankle and foot or twisting the pelvis.

If this feels uncomfortable you can always put your foot on a telephone directory, to actually lift the foot which remains on the ground slightly higher.

Do each stretch twice on each leg, alternating sides.

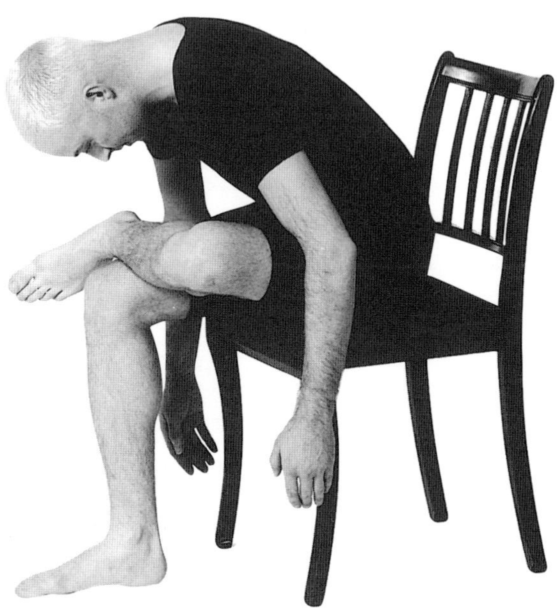

Exercise 5.

Hip Flexor and Front of the Thigh Exercise

You want to stretch the front of your thigh, the quadriceps muscle.

WATCHPOINT

Don't kneel on a hard floor as you may hurt your knee. With any exercises involving the knees, if you have any knee pain at any time, stop. Pain in the knee is contraindicated in any exercise.

In this lunge position, holding on to a chair to stabilize your weight, have one foot in front of you with the knee bent. The knee should be directly above the ankle. If the foot is behind the knee, you may strain your knee. You can either have the toes pointing directly forward or at '10 to 2' – think of your foot as a clock hand – whatever feels more comfortable for you. Due to the way in which your lower leg is aligned, the position of comfort may vary. Kneeling on the other leg, the foot behind you, very gently pull your stomach in. Press your hips forward and feel a stretch down the front of the thigh. At no point arch your back. Your stomach is pulled in, your shoulders are relaxed – imagine that someone has one hand on your stomach gently pushing your stomach in and the other hand on your bottom, which is being gently pushed forward to stabilize your spine.

The harder version of this exercise is simply to take your hands away from the chair, put them on your knee and take slightly more of a lean back to get a stronger stretch, but not at the expense of arching your back, straining your knee or letting your stomach protrude.

Repeat the exercise twice on each side, alternating legs.

1

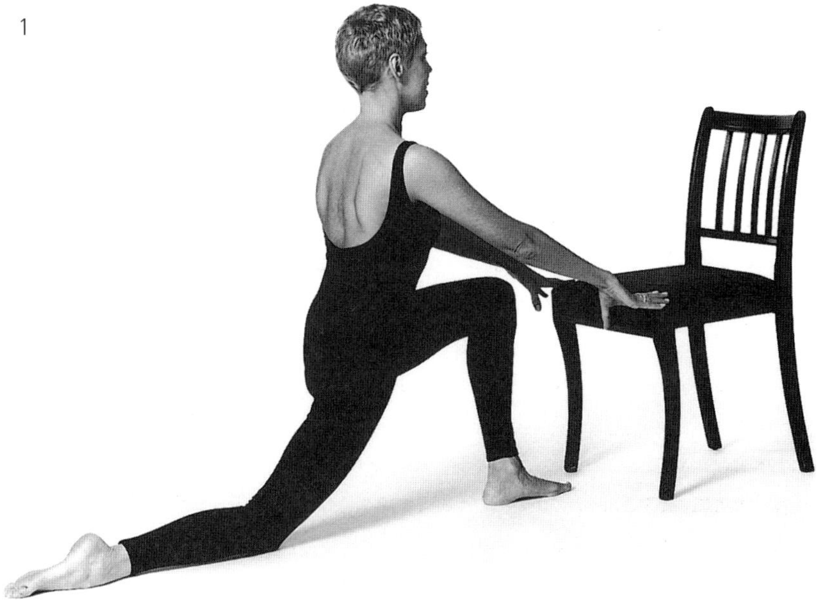

2

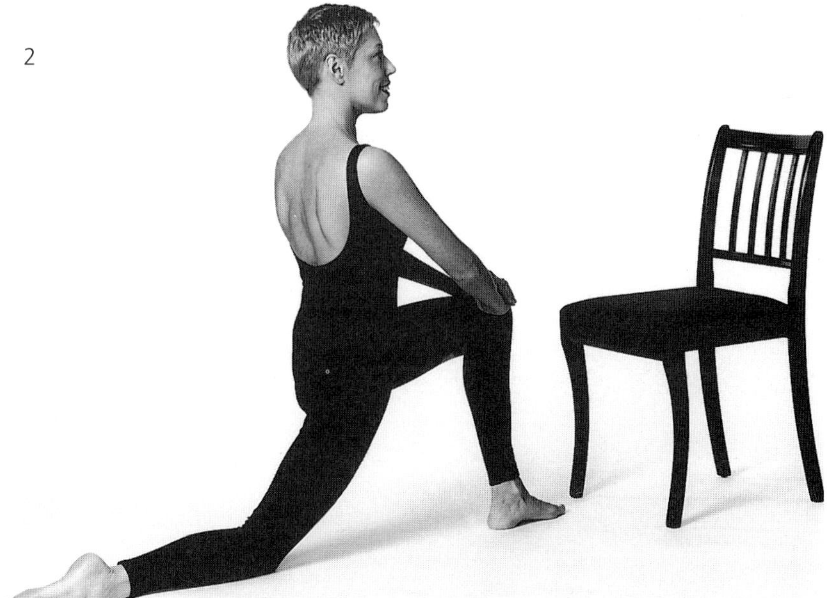

Thigh and buttock trimmer

Exercise 6.

Hamstring Stretch for the Back of the Leg

For this exercise, most people need to place a towel beneath the head.

Start with both feet on the floor, making sure you have equal weight down through both feet. The arms are beside you and the pelvis is in the correct position. Very gently bend your right knee into the chest. Grasp the back of your thigh with your left hand. Grasp the back of your calf with your right hand and gently unfold, straightening that leg with a flexed foot, and ease the leg towards you.

You'll know if you are doing it wrong if your bottom lifts. If this is impossible, instead of using your hands take a towel, place it around your calf and ease the leg towards you, keeping your neck and shoulders relaxed.

Do the right, then the left leg, and repeat – a minimum of twice on each side, holding for 30 seconds.

WATCHPOINT

Don't pull on your leg so that your bottom leaves the floor as your pelvis will twist. You want to flex the foot without overly tensing the feet and gently straighten that knee. It is more important to get the knee straighter than to bring the leg closer to you.

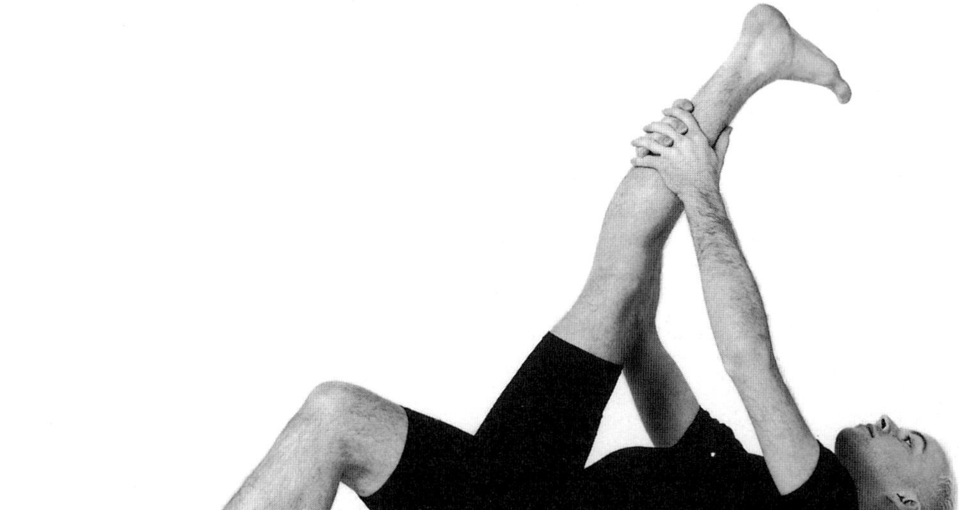

Thigh and buttock trimmer

Pilates homework

Helen Barnes, a make-up artist, began Pilates in January, 1998, because she was looking for an exercise programme that would make her body long, lean and strong. She really liked the idea that she could obtain these results without the pain of going to the gym.

'I used to get back problems from carrying heavy bags of equipment up and down the stairs in airports, when I was working. I pulled my back out every week and I'd then be in pain for two weeks. It was really awful. I'd go to the osteopath once or twice a month. My upper back was in terrible pain.

'Pilates has been enormously helpful. I used to have a stiff back as well. My lower spine was really rigid and I was not at all flexible. I had very little movement and was severely restricted. The Pilates exercises I was doing started to loosen up my spine. There are many exercises in Pilates in which you roll up and down with your back. Pilates also works on strengthening the weaker muscles. That is exactly what happened with my back – the weaker muscles started to get stronger.

'When I couldn't attend class twice a week at the Body Maintenance Studio, I made a point of doing Pilates at home. When you work at home you have to be very disciplined. You can't be lazy. Pilates, for me, is like an intellectual exercise. You have to really concentrate and isolate the muscles or the stretch on which you are working. If you do that correctly, it is really effective as there is nothing that is haphazard about Pilates. It requires precision, proper breathing and visualization.'

15-Minute Pilates

'I also learned to do some of the exercises from Lesley's first book, *15-Minute Pilates*. The exercises are simply explained and there are 'Watchpoints', so I could be aware of the incorrect movements I might do.

'Since I've begun Pilates, I haven't been to an osteopath. I can lift my heavy bags of equipment needed for work, but I have also taken a practical approach to the loads I must carry. Instead of a back pack I use a wheelie bag.

'I believe that due to Pilates, my body looks better. My thighs have reduced and my buttocks have trimmed down. I'm 34, and my body looks better now than when I was 20 when I swam and cycled regularly. Pilates is the only exercise programme I've stuck with. I've got bored with the gym, and bored with swimming. I think I'll do Pilates for the rest of my life.'

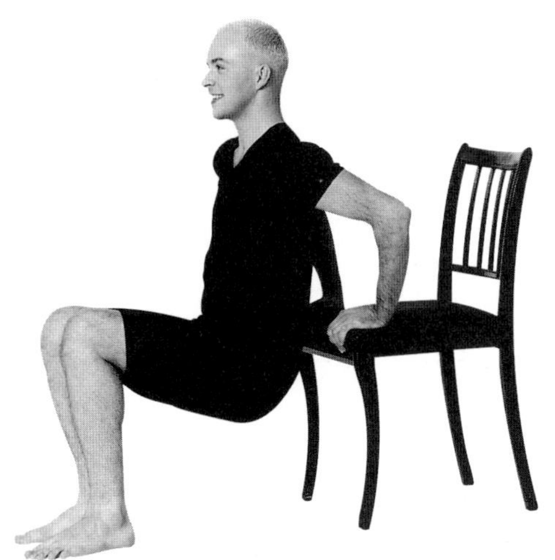

Step 7

A beautiful upper back – strength and definition

The spine is the central structure of the body. Tight or weak back muscles will eventually lead to problems. Taking steps to strengthen one's back is insurance for the future. A strong back and centre go hand in hand to present an upright and confident person.

In my experience as a Pilates teacher, all women want a beautiful upper back, gorgeous shoulders, lovely arms and triceps. The first four exercises will tone, condition and strengthen. Press-Ups and Dips are full-body exercises which will tone the body quite rapidly. The last three exercises are stretches which are absolutely essential after performing upper body work. Proper stretching will prevent you from having rounded shoulders and tight muscles. You want the most erotic upper body in the world: long, lean, and well toned. You can get away with a lot if you have beautiful upper shoulders and arms.

Exercise 1.
Press-Ups

This exercise is a slight variation of a Press-Up, which I use a great deal in my studio.

On your hands and knees you make a square with the body. Again, it is better not to kneel on a hard surface – use a towel or an exercise mat. To begin, knees are under the hips; the hands are under the shoulders. Cross one hand over the other. The neck is in line. There is no arching the back, the stomach is pulled in.

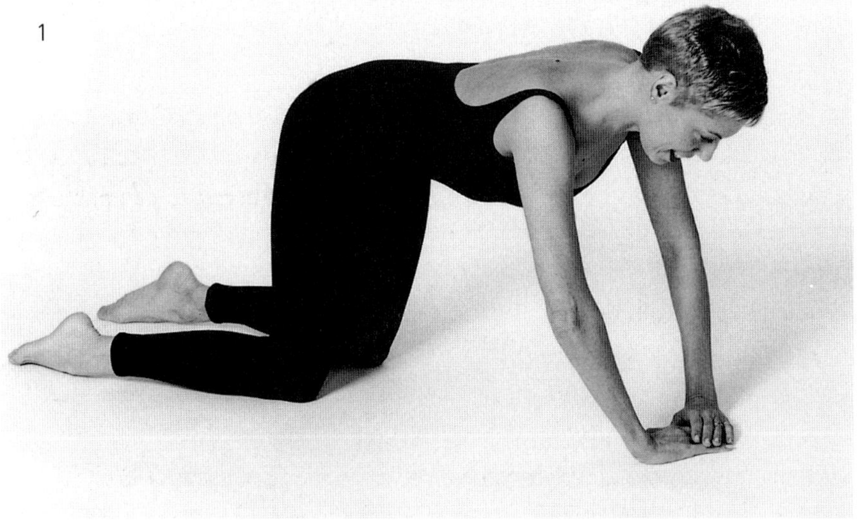
1

In this position, very gently, working with your entire body, tip yourself slightly forward over the arms. This does not mean you should arch your back. It is very natural, when assuming the press-up positions, to allow your head to drop. However, try to keep the head in a natural position, neither forward nor backward (photograph 2).

2

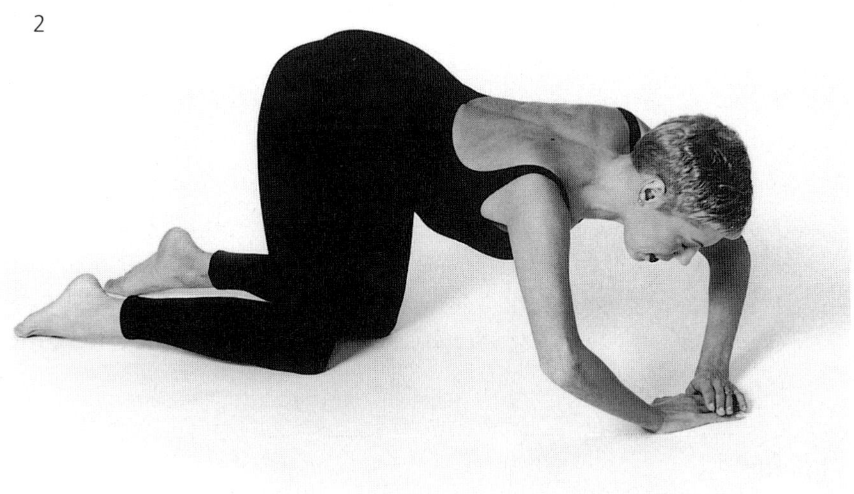

Begin by doing six repetitions – right hand on top, then the left, work up to an equal set of 10 or 12 with each hand on top. Very gently breathe in as you bend the arms, bringing the chest down. Breathe out as you push away.

WATCHPOINT

Do not lock the elbows.

If it is possible, do the Press-Ups in front of a mirror. Thus, when you press down, your head should not lower and your chin should not stick out. When you start this exercise you will feel your weight rocking slightly forwards and backwards. Try to stabilize the weight over the arms so that you get the most strengthening through the upper back, the shoulders and all the muscles in the arms – the triceps and biceps. You will be both strengthening and toning. This will not only result in a great-looking upper body, but you will be generating some upper-body strength as well. If you can't easily open your own bottle of champagne, then you have a problem.

Exercise 2.

Dips

Most women find Dips difficult to start with because of the lack of strength in the backs of their arms.

Using a chair placed against a wall for support, have your hands wide enough so that your shoulders don't feel pinched together. Fingers are facing forward. Make sure in this position that your knees are over your ankles. If they're not you'll be using your thighs as opposed to the backs of your arms.

1

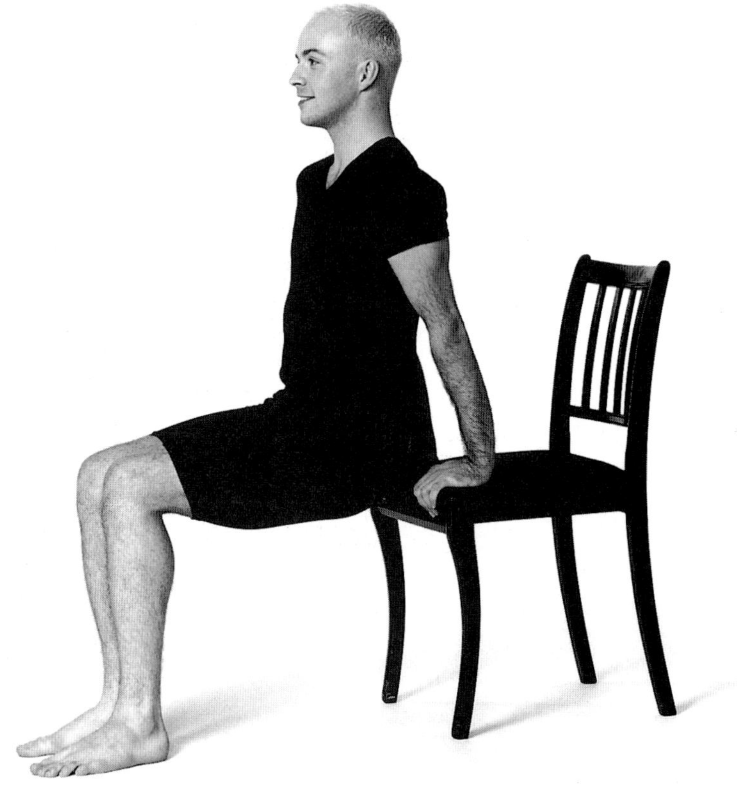

As you breathe in, you bend, as you breathe out, you straighten.

Make sure as you do the Dips that you're sliding your bottom down the edge of the chair and that you're not sliding forward, as the body will automatically prefer to do, and take the strain in the front of the thighs.

You might only be able to start with eight repetitions – gently build up to 25. You can do two sets, alternating one set of Press-Ups and one set of Dips.

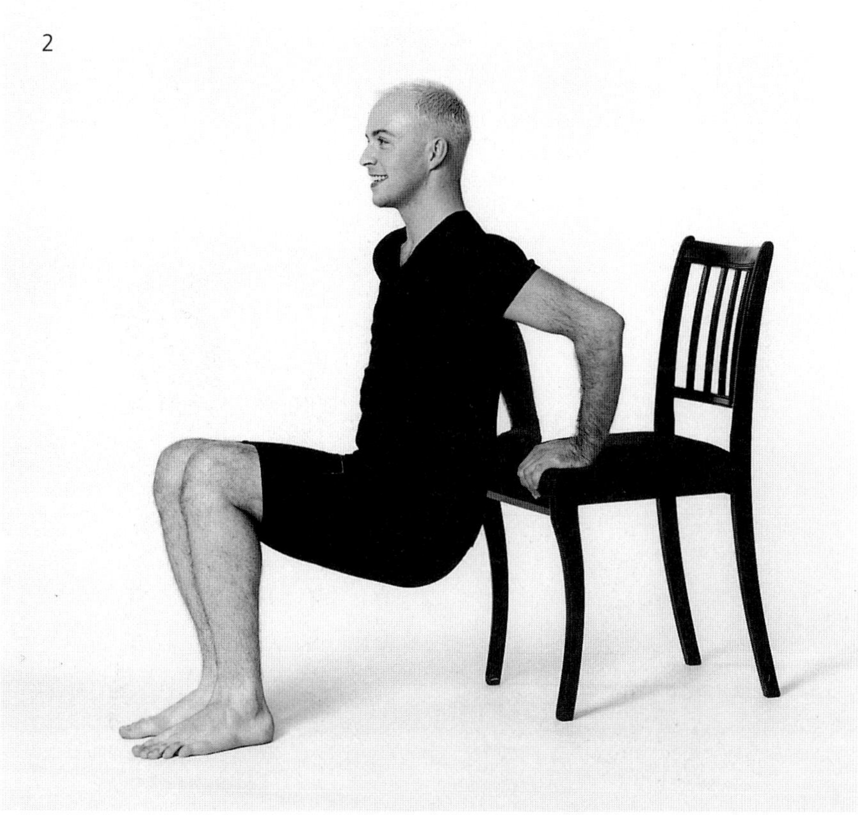

Exercise 3.
Triceps Strengthening

These require the use of a Dynaband, a long piece of elasticized rubber available at most health and fitness stores. Dynabands come in different weights and are colour-coded. Sit up straight, shoulders relaxed – do not arch your back. When working with a Dynaband you must gauge the length of your arms so that you have a reasonable amount of tension in the band. Wrap the Dynaband around your hands and hold it between them. There should not be much more than a 3 feet (1 metre) between the two hands. Obviously, if you have tight or rounded shoulders you might want to loosen the Dynaband at the start.

Place your right hand on your left shoulder. Lift the left elbow as high as you can without lifting the shoulder.

1

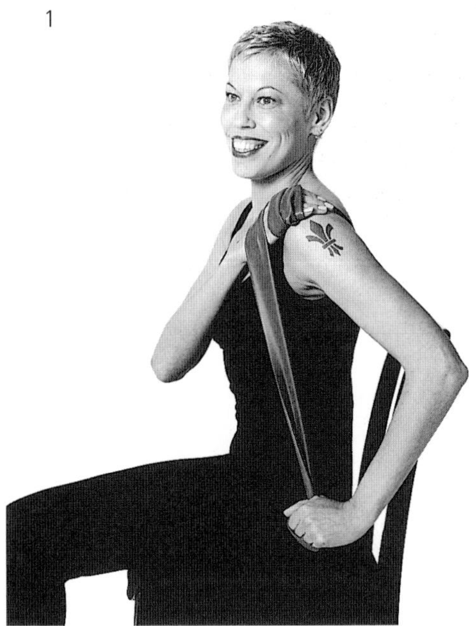

Keep that elbow high, and squeeze to straighten. Do 15 repetitions on each arm, and do two or three sets.

WATCHPOINT

Keep the elbow close to the body, don't let the shoulders lift. Try to keep the elbow stable and not allow it to lock.

2

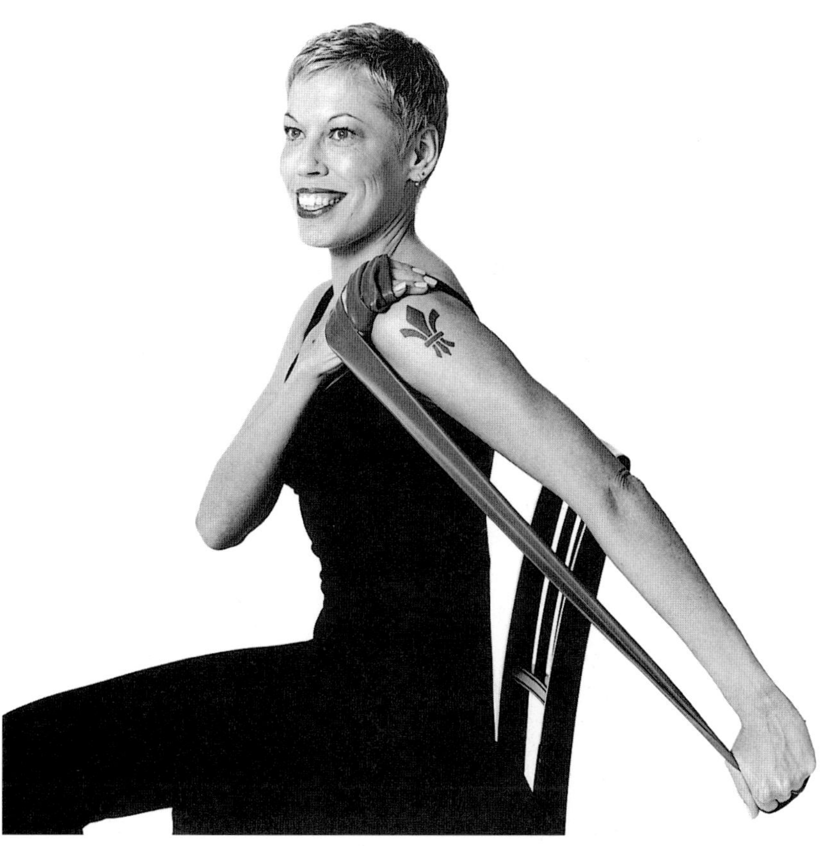

Exercise 4.
Strengthening the Pecs

Pecs are muscles that help support a woman's breasts. This is another exercise which is good to do in front of a mirror. Sitting on a chair, make sure you're not arching forward or backward, weight solidly placed over both feet. Feel as if you are sitting back into yourself slightly, without sinking. The stomach is pulled in and up but you will also instinctively want to sit forward slightly. If you have any doubts, do the exercise sitting on a chair which has a back, in order to support the middle of your back.

Again, you want to have the Dynaband so there is about 3 feet (1 metre) between your hands, but in this case the distance can be slightly less than this. Holding the Dynaband in front of you, hands facing down, look in the mirror to check that your shoulders are down and the arms are at chest level. Breathe out, keeping the elbows slightly soft, neither bent nor straight. Very gently pull. You may feel a stretch across your chest and your arms will be toned as well.

Repeat 10 times, or build up to three sets of 10.

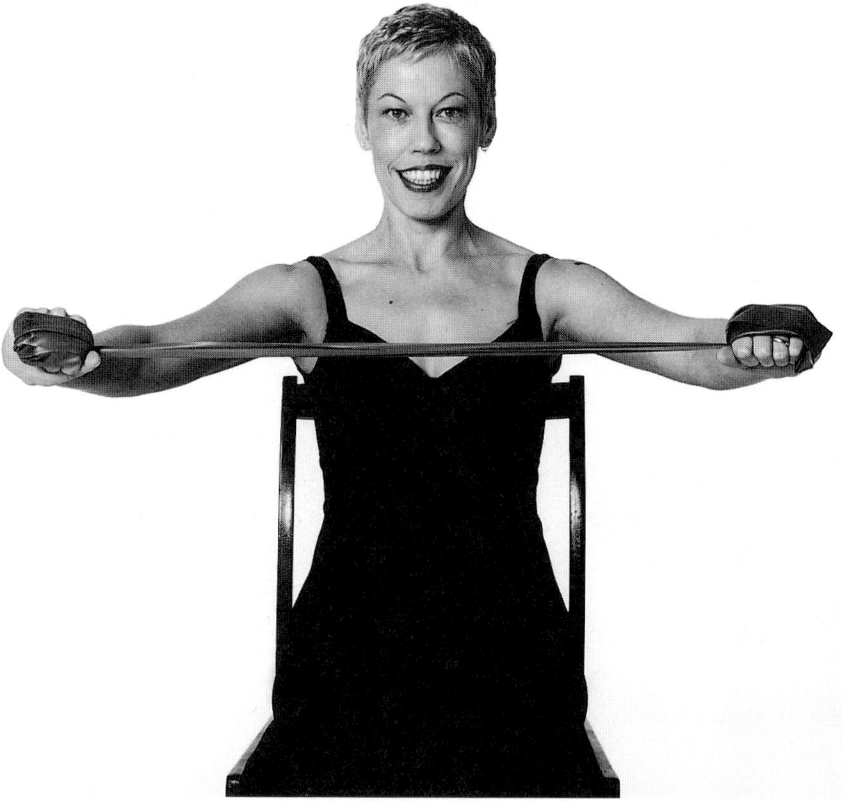

A beautiful upper back – strength and definition

Exercise 5.

Shoulder Stretch (1)

This exercise can be done with either a towel or a Dynaband. Sitting on a chair, all the same rules apply: stomach in, shoulders down. Very gently start with the Dynaband or towel at the hips.

1

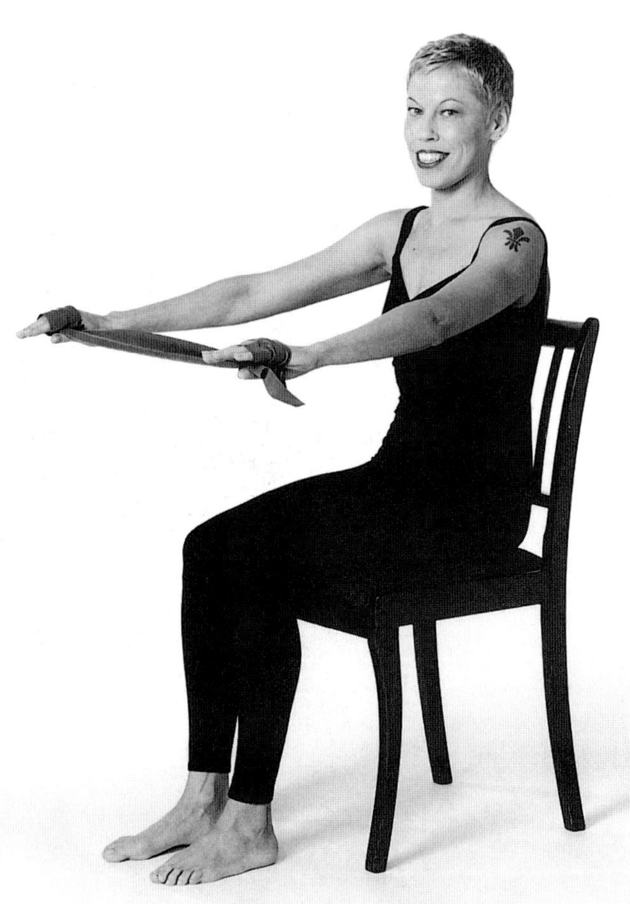

Breathe in and lift the towel to the crown of the head.

Breathe out and pull the towel down so that it just touches the head. Breathe in and straighten, breathe out and bring the towel forward and down.

Do 10 repetitions.

WATCHPOINT

Don't arch the back and don't take the towel too far back. If you have a problem with this, do it seated with your back against the wall to support your middle back. Again, the elbows are slightly forward in your peripheral vision. Thus, when you bend the arms and bring the towel down you can see your elbows without moving your head.

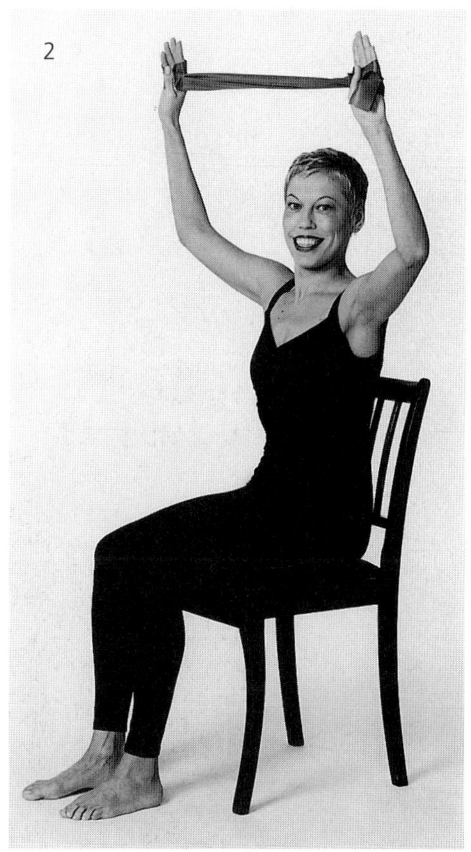

Shoulder Stretch (2)

Assume the same position as in the previous exercise. Holding the towel in front, level with the chest, very carefully twist one way until you've made a pole. Breathe in, breathe out, twist the other way, to stretch your shoulders.

Do 10 repetitions.

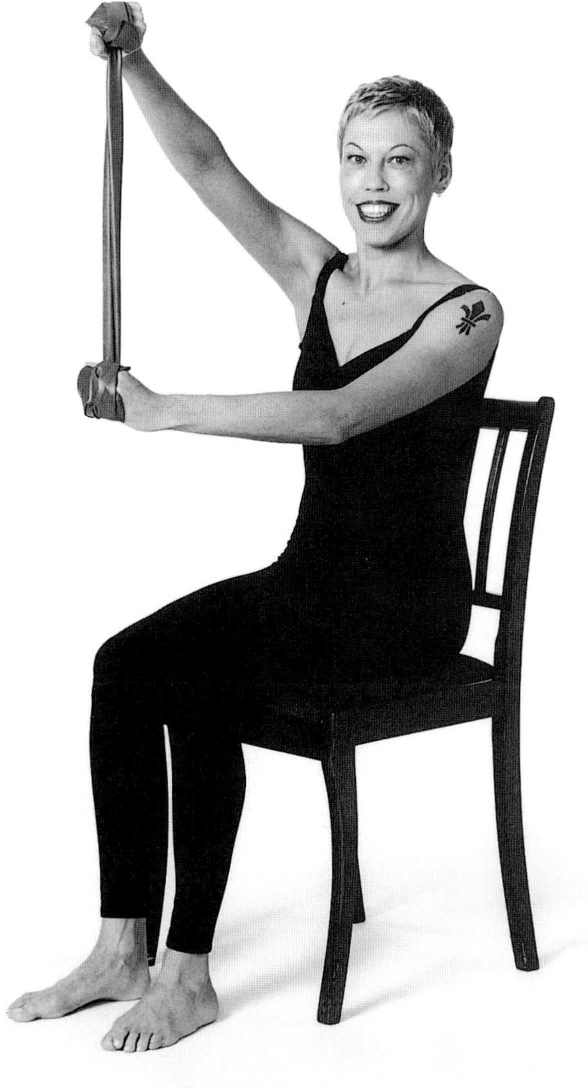

A beautiful upper back – strength and definition

Shoulder Stretch (3)

Leaning against a wall, have the arms as wide apart as possible, and place the palms on the wall. The feet are on the floor, hip-width apart. The stomach is in, the tailbone is dropped. The ears are between the arms. Do not allow the head to go either forward or backward. You'll know if you do, as you will feel a strain in the neck.

As you breathe out gently press your chest towards the wall as the hands slide up the wall. Try to stretch up as far as you can.

Do 10 repetitions.

WATCHPOINT

Make sure the stomach is in, don't arch your back, and be sure that both heels stay on the floor.

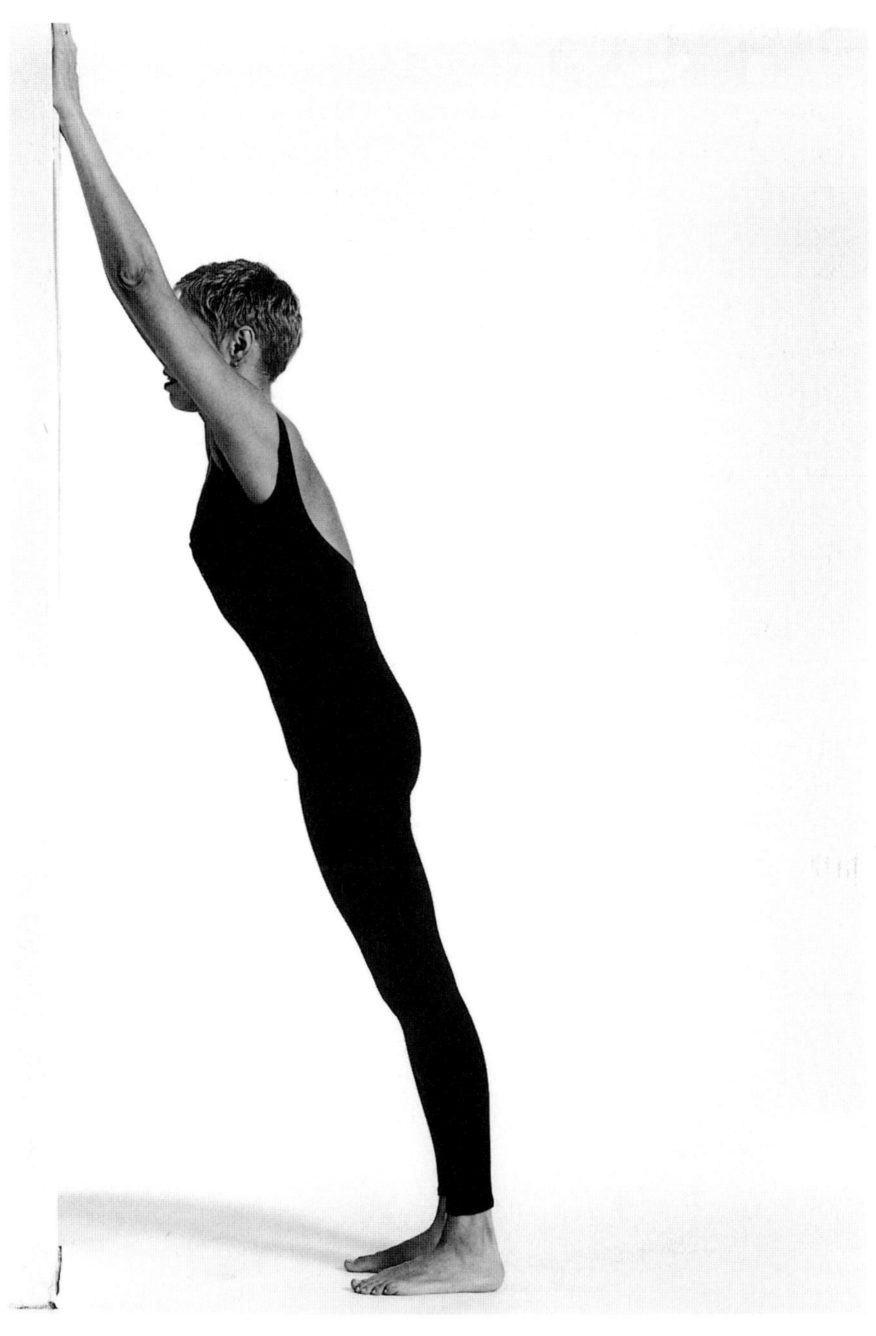

A beautiful upper back – strength and definition

Shoulder mobility

Daryl Bennett was out shopping one day and for no apparent reason his back went into spasm. 'It scared me to death. I immediately went home and called Thomas [Paton]. He told me what position to get into and how better to relieve the pain I was in.'

Lying on the floor, with his feet on a sofa, Daryl kept his back as still as possible and also kept it warm. Then Lesley Ackland phoned. Lesley, Thomas and Daryl are all good friends. Daryl remembers:

'Lesley was just asking me to move in different ways and to describe what I felt. She was virtually able to analyse what was wrong over the phone. Having somebody talk me through it was enormously helpful and reassuring. Afterwards she said I should come to the Body Maintenance Studio.

'I knew Pilates had helped Thomas with his dance injuries, but it had never occurred to me to go to Body Maintenance myself. Lesley's phone call changed that. For the first time I understood that I could really benefit from attending her classes.'

Long Hours

'Through the spasm, my body was telling me it was time to do something about bad posture, to try and correct all the bad habits that I had picked up. As a director of an incoming tour company, which brings Americans to the UK and arranges their travel needs, I work long hours in front of a computer.

'The initial Pilates exercises helped to strengthen my stomach, which I hardly use during the day. As a result, my back was being put under unnecessary strain.

'My routine also included exercises to increase my shoulder mobility. These also helped to correct my posture. Because I spend all day hunched over a keyboard, I had become terribly round-shouldered. Lesley is trying to open up my shoulders and give me a wider chest without actually building muscle. Due to Pilates I now have both better posture and alignment.

'When I do press-ups, I try to concentrate on maintaining the space between the sternum and edge of the shoulders, and the spine and the shoulder blades.'

Better Body Shape

'After five months of doing Pilates, change has come quickly. I have a better body shape. I have broader, more mobile shoulders and a better-defined stomach. I've actually got stomach muscles now that I've never had before. Pilates has improved my posture and, just as importantly, made me think about my posture more. Obviously I can't constantly be thinking about the way I'm sitting at work because work takes over. On occasion, however, I deliberately take the time and attempt to sit up and improve the way I'm key-boarding.

'I am now aware that the way you hold yourself throughout the day can help relieve any area of weakness that you might have. If you have a weak back, which I do, then sitting upright and using the stomach muscles to support myself, rather than slouching in my chair, is going to alleviate any stress or strain I am putting on my back as a result of bad posture.

'After another week of Pilates you see another change, flattening of the stomach, thinning of the waist, a broadening of the shoulders. It is an incentive to keep going until you have the perfect body for you, as Lesley keeps telling us. Pilates is not a tiring exercise regime. It's not boring. It's something to look forward to. In fact I overheard someone in the studio say, "It's an oasis of calm at the end of the week".'

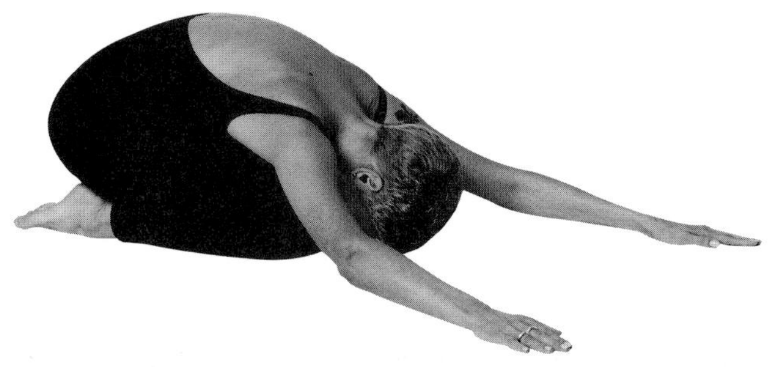

Step 8

A beautiful lower back – strength and stability

You cannot stand upright if you have a tight, weak back. Any minor adjustments which you yourself make to try and correct the way in which you walk, sit and stand will only create further problems. Gentle exercise and control are the key. If you envision the exercises in Step 8 as stomach exercises, you can't go wrong. If you think of them as back exercises the result will be frenetic movement that won't accomplish much except possibly 'concertina-ing' your bones.

If time allows, these lower back exercises should be done after the stomach exercises. These exercises work better as a pair. You must strengthen your stomach before you start working on your back, as the abdominal muscles initiate the work needed to develop a strong back. All exercises are directed from the abdominals.

Exercise 1.
Pelvic Tilt

This exercise is done with your heels on a chair. Lie on your back with your head on a towel or a cushion, the arms beside you. You are near or far enough away from the chair so that your tailbone is weighted on the mat.

Before you do anything else, relax and allow your spine to settle into its natural position. The chin is slightly dropped forward and shoulders are relaxed.

This is another exercise in which you inhale to prepare and exhale on the point of effort. As you breathe out, you tip the pelvis forward and you very gently roll up from the base of the spine one vertebra at a time until you are just below your shoulder blades. If you feel your ribs sticking forward or your neck shortening you'll know you've gone too far. Inhale at the top, then exhale through your upper back until your tailbone reaches the floor.

WATCHPOINT

Legs stay in parallel, grip your bottom as little as possible.

There is a good chance you will feel this in your calf and hamstrings. Don't worry about this unless it is really uncomfortable. If this is the case, skip this exercise.

There is a more difficult version of this exercise. Instead of having your palms on the floor, you are resting on your elbows. This is harder because you have a less stable base throughout the upper body. Don't be tempted to push too high.

Do approximately 10 repetitions.

1

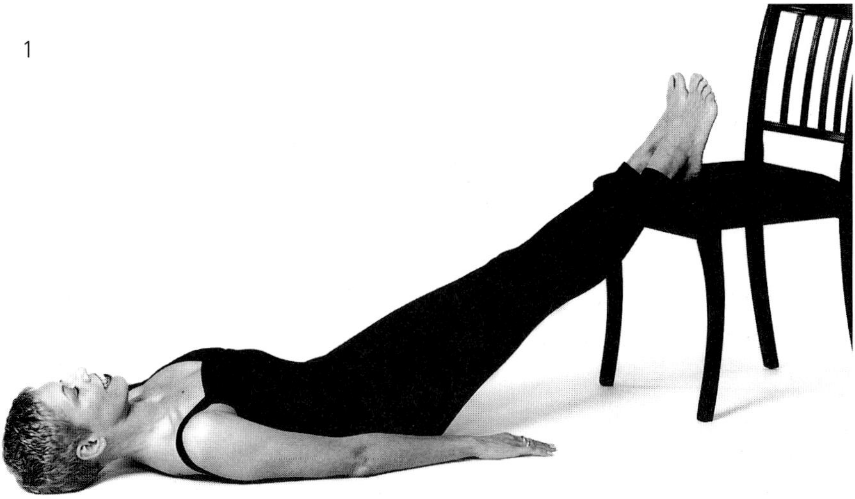

2

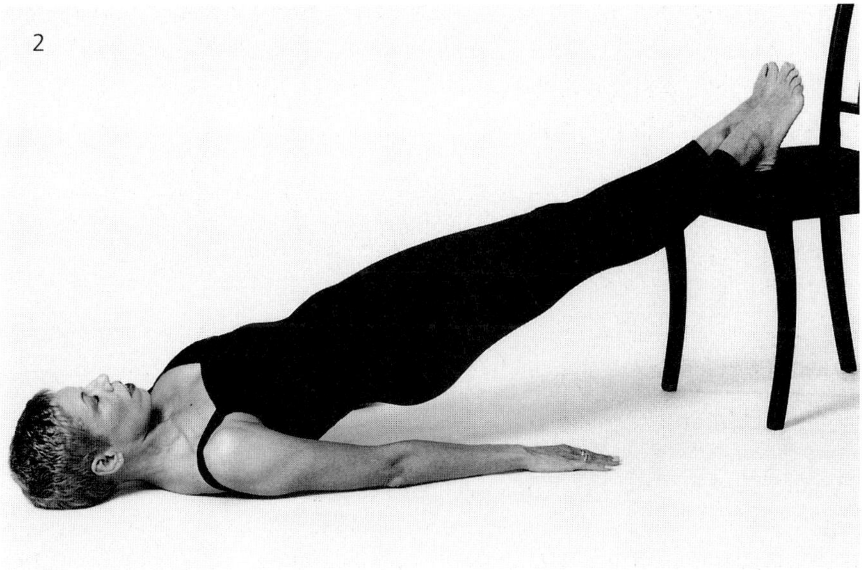

Exercise 2.
Back Strengthener (1)

These are dynamic exercises, which use the arms without over-arching the back. Initially the movement comes from the stomach. The back then takes over and strengthens.

Lie on your stomach with your feet apart, forehead resting on the floor. Take the arms as wide as you can without feeling your shoulder blades pinching together. Before you start, breathe in, feel your stomach drop to the floor. Breathe out, pull your stomach into your spine and relax your tailbone.

1

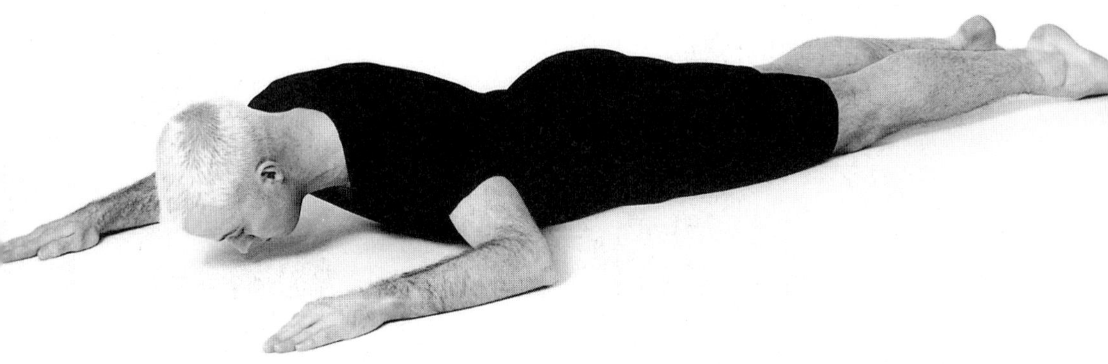

Don't lift the head separately. Keep it in line and focus on the same point for the duration of the exercise. Breathe out and gently press down into the arms, feel the stomach and chest leaving the mat, the elbows staying on the mat. Pause, breathe in and lower.

The buttocks will contract slightly, but try hard to keep them relaxed. The buttocks and the hamstrings have to work minimally, but you must keep them as relaxed as possible and use the stomach as the instigator of the exercise. If you feel your back pinching, you've gone too far. If you feel any strain in the neck you've taken the head too far back. Repeat 10 times.

2

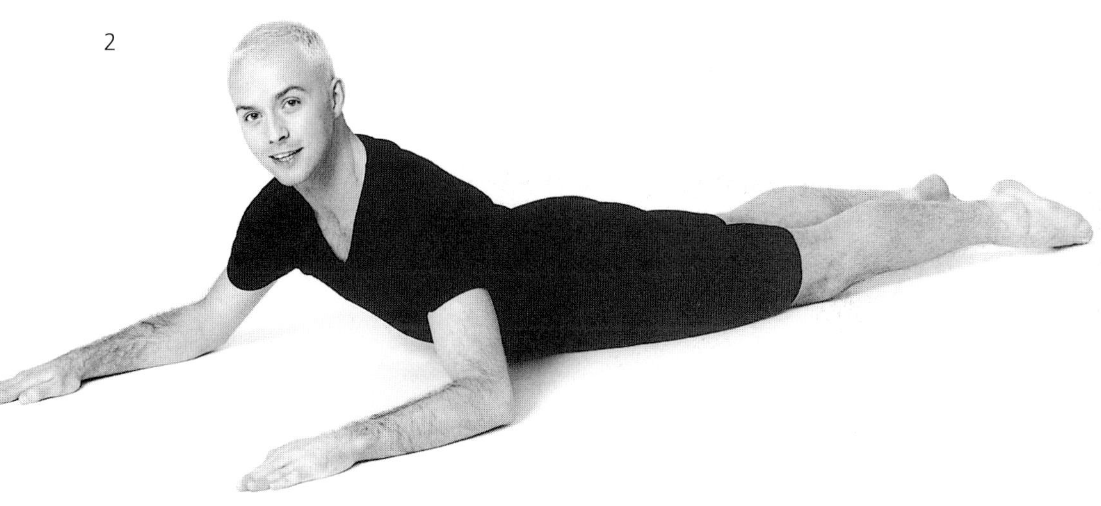

Exercise 3.
Back Strengthener (2)

The variation on this exercise is a stronger version of the previous exercise. Breathe out, gently press down into the arms, feel the stomach, chest and then the elbows leaving the mat. Breathe in and relax down to the floor.

You should start off with 5 repetitions and slowly increase the number to 10.

WATCHPOINT

Shoulders don't lift and the lumbar spine – the lower back – doesn't 'concertina' together.

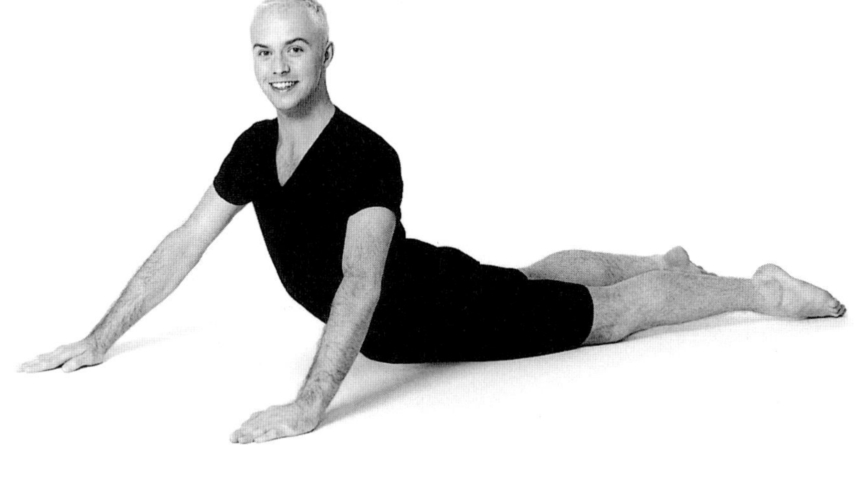

A beautiful lower back – strength and stability

Exercise 4.

Back Strengthener (3)

All the same rules apply as in the previous exercise, except in this case the arms are beside you. In this exercise do not go as high, do not lock the elbows and do not let the head tip forward or back. With your arms beside you, your forehead on the ground, you breathe out. The stomach goes in and your chest and shoulders gently float. If the exercise develops into a heave, you're not strong enough to do it.

You should start off with 5 repetitions and slowly build up to 10.

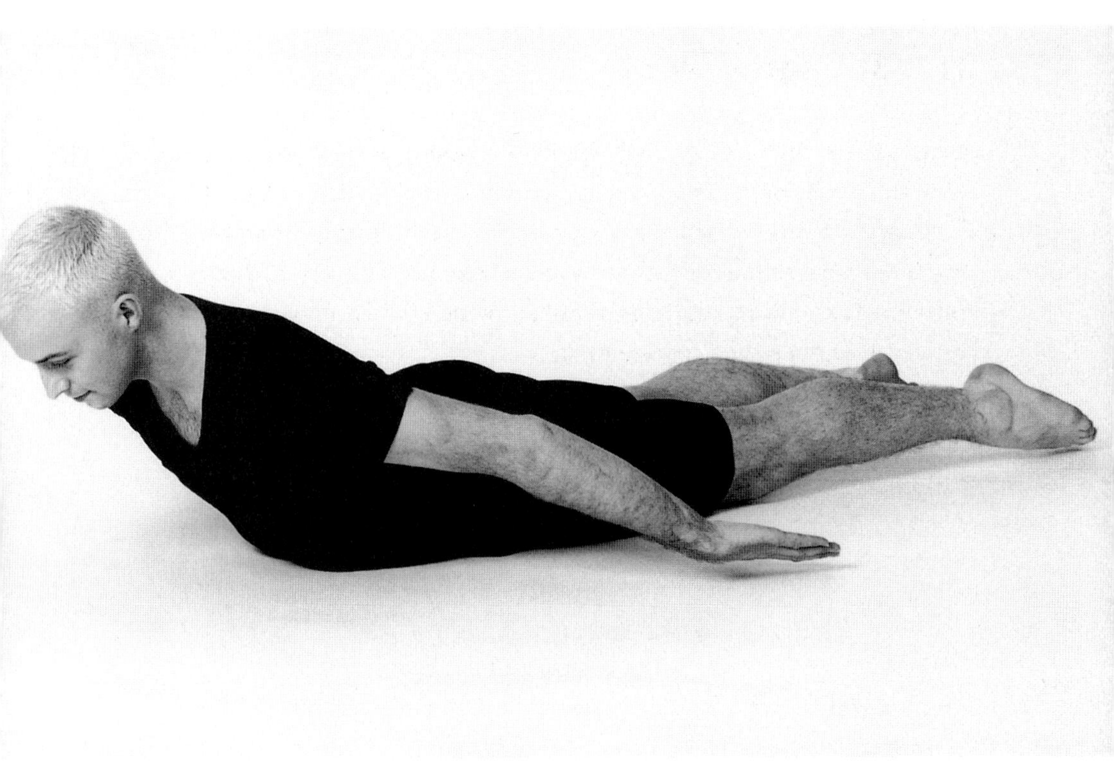

Whether you do one or six of the back exercises in this sequence, you should finish on The Child's Relaxation Pose. Many people aren't strong enough to do the Advanced Back Exercises and they will stop at Back Strengthener 3. Therefore, regardless of the order in which the exercises are performed, one should finish with The Child's Relaxation Pose (see page 158).

Advanced Back Exercises 5 & 6

These exercises are more difficult because they are full-bodyweight exercises. As well as being both stomach- and back-strengthening exercises, they will also tone the upper body – the shoulders, arms and wrists.

If your wrists are exceptionally tight these exercises will be too hard for you. If you find these exercises uncomfortable, don't do them.

Sit on the ground, back straight, with your legs in front of you. Place the hands on either side of you. As you breathe out gently push down into the floor and straighten the elbows; hold for a count of three and gently lower.

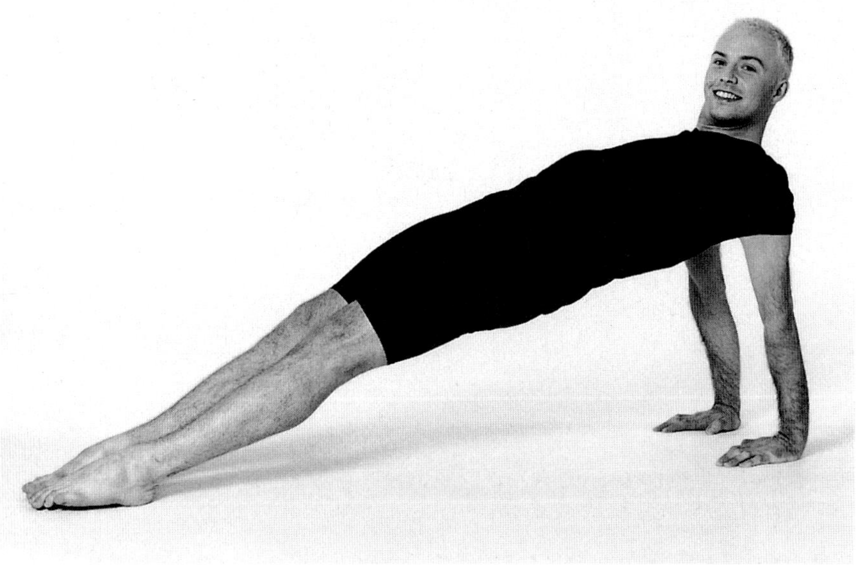

Don't lock the elbows, don't let the chin drop forward or back. Don't push so high that you can feel your hips thrusting forward, your buttocks pinching too tightly or your lower back contracting. Do 5 repetitions and build up to 10.

A much harder version is as follows: After you've lifted, hold the position, keeping the pelvis completely stable. Breathe in and lift one leg, breathe out to lower. Repeat with the other leg. Lower your buttocks to the floor and repeat four more times, slowly building up the exercise as you get stronger.

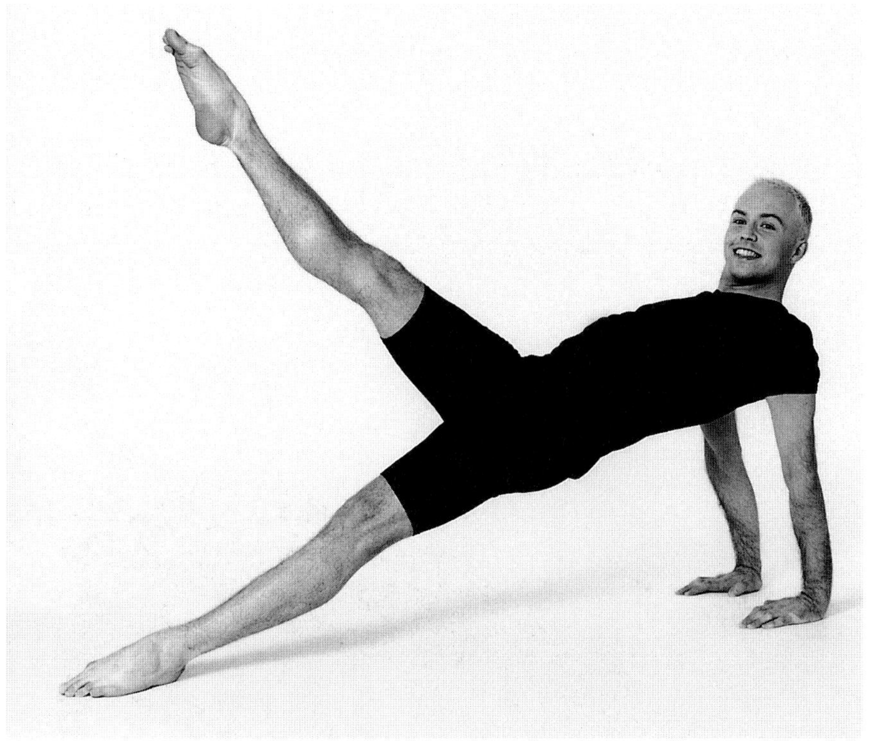

You'll know if the exercise is uncomfortable. Your wrist and upper back will feel sore. In the beginning you might not be strong enough to do the exercise but you will become stronger by doing the first four exercises in this section.

Exercise 7.
The Child's Relaxation Pose

Sit back with your bottom on your heels, your arms in front of you, and just relax. Count to between 10 and 30 seconds. Then, looking at the floor, very gently roll up one vertebra at a time and come up to a seated position.

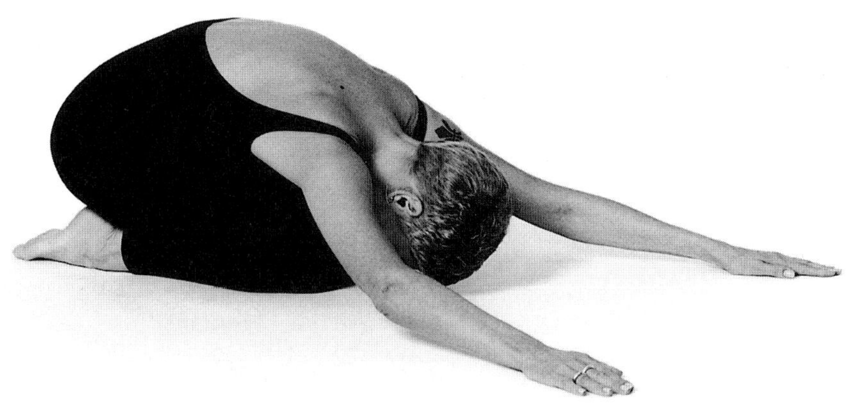

The Child's Relaxation Pose should be used at the end of the exercise sequence.

I pick up my own napkins, thank you

Julie Myerson is a novelist and literary critic.

'Some time in my mid-twenties, my lower back began to seize up without warning. At worst, I was in agony, barely able to move. At best, just crooked, in permanent, grumbling discomfort.

'At first, the problem was easily put right by a single visit to an osteopath. But five years and three pregnancies later, I had endured more acute episodes than I could count and a day rarely passed without pain.

'Otherwise fit and energetic, I could not lift my kids on to a swing without risking three days in bed. Back sufferers are bores: they live in fear of triggering the pain and, cruel but true, the fear itself becomes a trigger. I was habitually tense, careful, resentfully resigned to a self-protective, no-fun-and-games attitude. At 32, I felt old.

'Orthopaedic surgeons scanned and prodded, but concluded that an operation was not appropriate. They told me I had scoliosis – an ominous, medieval torture chamber sort of word – and that it might "stabilize".

'In fact, scoliosis (curvature and twisting of the spine) affects about one in 250 of the population. My own is mild-ish, idiopathic (an expert's word, meaning the experts are not sure why it developed) and functional (caused by muscles). Pitifully weak back and stomach muscles – the results of pregnancy, as well as years of maniacally self-protective behaviour – had not helped.

'I tried acupuncture, yoga, hypnotherapy, the Alexander technique – all positive, all helpful, but only for about three weeks. The amount of money I had chucked at my spine by now was becoming depressing.

'Lesley Ackland was the third Pilates teacher I had tried. From the start, she was encouragingly uncompromising. "You've got to be able to use your body confidently and spontaneously," she told me. "What if you're in a restaurant and you drop your napkin? You've got to be able to pick it up just like that, without thinking."

'She promised to help realign my body, relax my posture and enable me to move with greater spontaneity. "Apart from anything else," she said, "a scoliosis isn't glamorous." I liked the way she was thinking.

'The first thing she did was to devise a mobility and strengthening programme and a general fitness routine, with emphasis on the abdomen, lower back and legs, to tackle my upper back scoliosis. I agreed to exercise three times a week – a big commitment, but one that has since paid off. Work was also begun on my feet and lower legs which were hopelessly misaligned and responsible for a gait that did not help my back.

'In any one session, I would do stomach and back strengthening on a mat on the floor, arm weights on a "barrel" and legwork with my feet in sprung straps or in the "plié machine" – a daunting-looking contraption on which I have to lie down and push away with my feet. I also exercise with a tennis ball, a slope, a "wobble board" and a large rubber physiotherapy ball.

'My progress, at first exhilaratingly swift, has since slowed to a realistic, but encouraging rate, but has never stopped. There are occasional setbacks (especially when a new movement has been introduced and my body reluctantly adapts), but I am straighter than I ever thought possible, my acute episodes are further and further apart and most days I am without pain.

'It is bewildering that no back specialist and few of the osteopaths I have encountered have heard of the Pilates method. For years I was sent home from my scans and tests with nothing but a sense of hopelessness.

'A year later, I cannot say I am cured but my problem has changed in a way I find both lasting and acceptable. I will probably never go out of my way to lift chubby toddlers, but I can walk for miles, run for a bus, sit and play with Lego on the floor, and stand at a party without suffering the next day.

'And the next time you see my napkin flutter to the floor, please do not pick it up for me.'

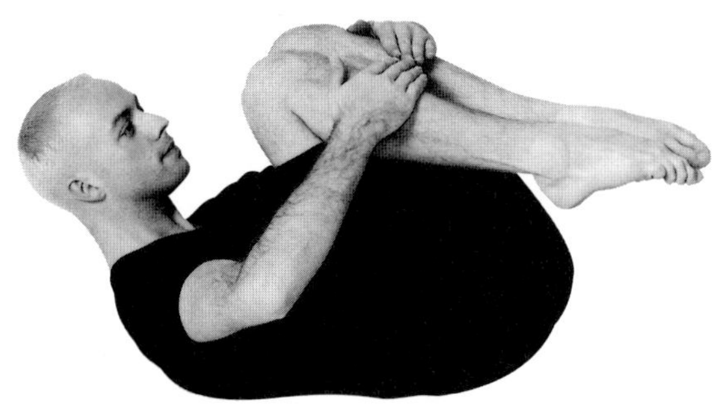

Step 9

Morning maintenance for bad backs

This 10-minute exercise programme is based on the exercises many of my clients who have had back injuries or who suffer from chronic back pain do first thing in the morning. It is a selection of six exercises to do in the morning between the time you get out of bed and go to work, which will basically strengthen and mobilize your lower back.

When you wake up in the morning with a bad back, you tend to feel quite immobile, stiff and uncomfortable. Your body doesn't want to move and you have difficulty even straightening up.

Exercise 1.

Pelvic Tilt

This is a basic Pelvic Tilt. Lie on a towel or mat. You may also need to place a small towel behind your head. The feet, hips and knees are all parallel, hip-width apart, the tailbone is relaxed on the mat without feeling forced down. The shoulders are relaxed and the neck is long. The arms are softly beside you.

Without gripping your bottom, very gently tip your pelvis upwards as you breathe out, breathe in and lower. This is a low pelvic tilt. You don't want to lift higher than your waist. You are only lifting your lower back off the ground. It is important to exhale as you lift. Breathe in, keeping your neck long, and roll all the way down.

Do approximately 10 repetitions.

Try to get that primary curve in your lower back working to warm up the lower back, bringing the blood supply into that area.

1

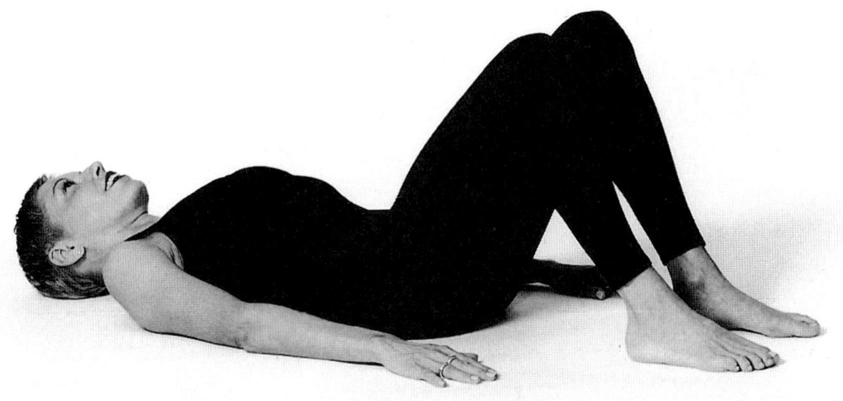

2

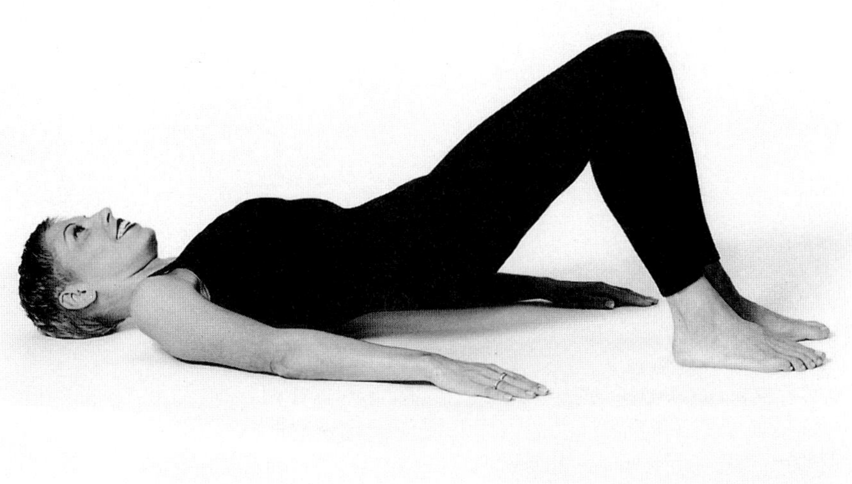

Exercise 2.

Passive Stretch for the Lower Back

Lie in the same position as for the previous exercise. This is a passive stretch for the lower back and the hamstrings. Very gently bend your right knee into your chest, holding on to the shin, below the kneecap. Have the elbows lifted to the side. You should not feel tension in your shoulders.

Breathe out and pull one knee into your chest, stretching the other leg along the floor and gently flexing both feet. You should feel a passive stretch going through the bent leg and buttock. You will also feel a hamstring and calf stretch going through the straight leg. Count: one, two, three, four. Then change sides.

10 repetitions altogether, alternating five on each leg.

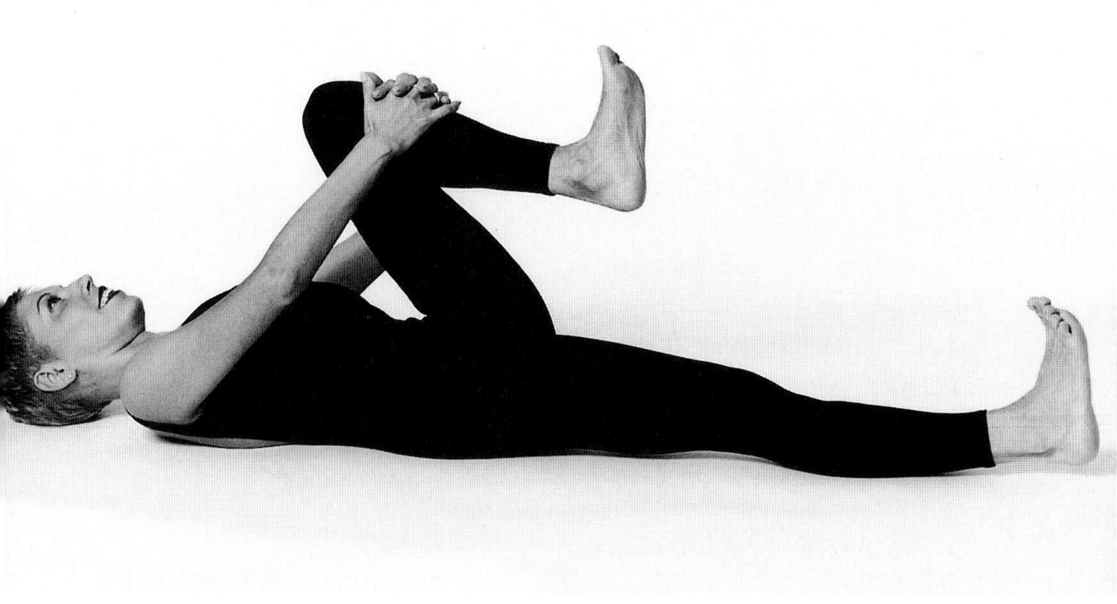

Morning maintenance for bad backs

Exercise 3.
Hip Roll

This mobilization exercise for the spine will warm up the back. It is a gentle stretch for the lower back and the hip. The stomach is the instigator of the movement. You are in exactly the same position as for the previous exercise, but this time you cross one leg over the other. It doesn't matter which leg you start with, but the other foot is firmly on the floor.

The arms are beside you, palms facing down below shoulder level. The stomach is the stabilizer in this exercise, and at no point does either shoulder blade leave the mat.

Breathe in, breathe out and take a gentle twist one way, looking away from the direction you are twisting. Come back to the original position. Breathe in from the centre, and breathe out as you twist in the opposite direction (photograph 2).

You'll know if you've gone too far, as your stomach will protrude and your shoulders will leave the mat. If it's too hard for you to move your head and look in the opposite direction due to coordination problems, start by looking directly up while you familiarize yourself with the exercise. When you're comfortable you can begin turning the head.

Do 10 twists with one leg on top, then 10 twists with the other.

1

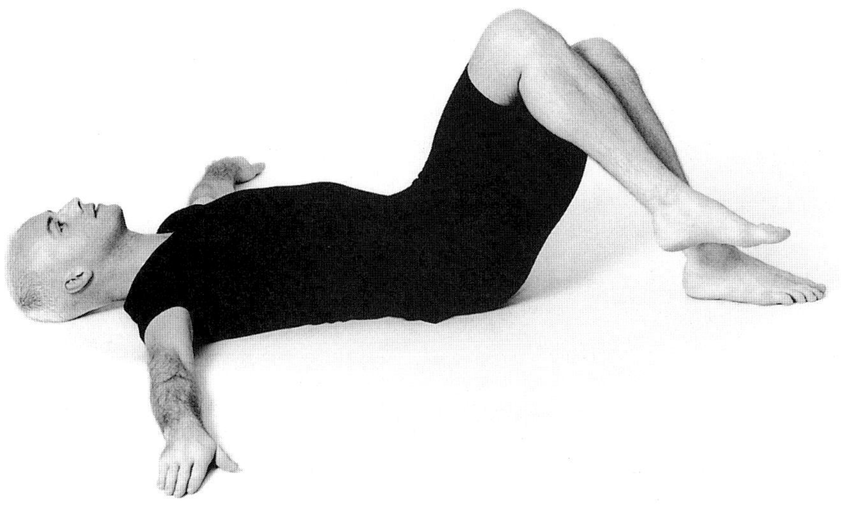

2

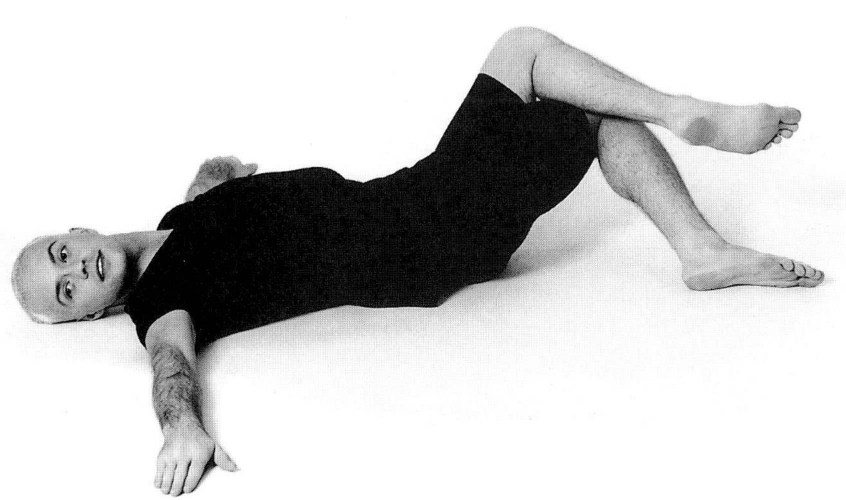

Exercise 4.

Basic Back of the Hip and Bottom Stretch

If you have a bad back, it is very likely that your buttock muscles and your hamstrings will be tight. Sit on the floor, or you may lean against a wall.

Stretch your left leg out in front of you. Cross your right foot over your left knee, keeping your right hand on the floor. Hold on to your right knee with your left hand, as you gently ease that knee into your chest. Then rotate your body around to the right. The left leg in front of you is parallel to the floor. Keep your foot to the ceiling and your shoulders relaxed. Don't let your foot roll out of line to the knee. Feel the stretch through your buttock.

Repeat four times, each time alternating legs and the direction you turn. Hold each stretch for 30 seconds.

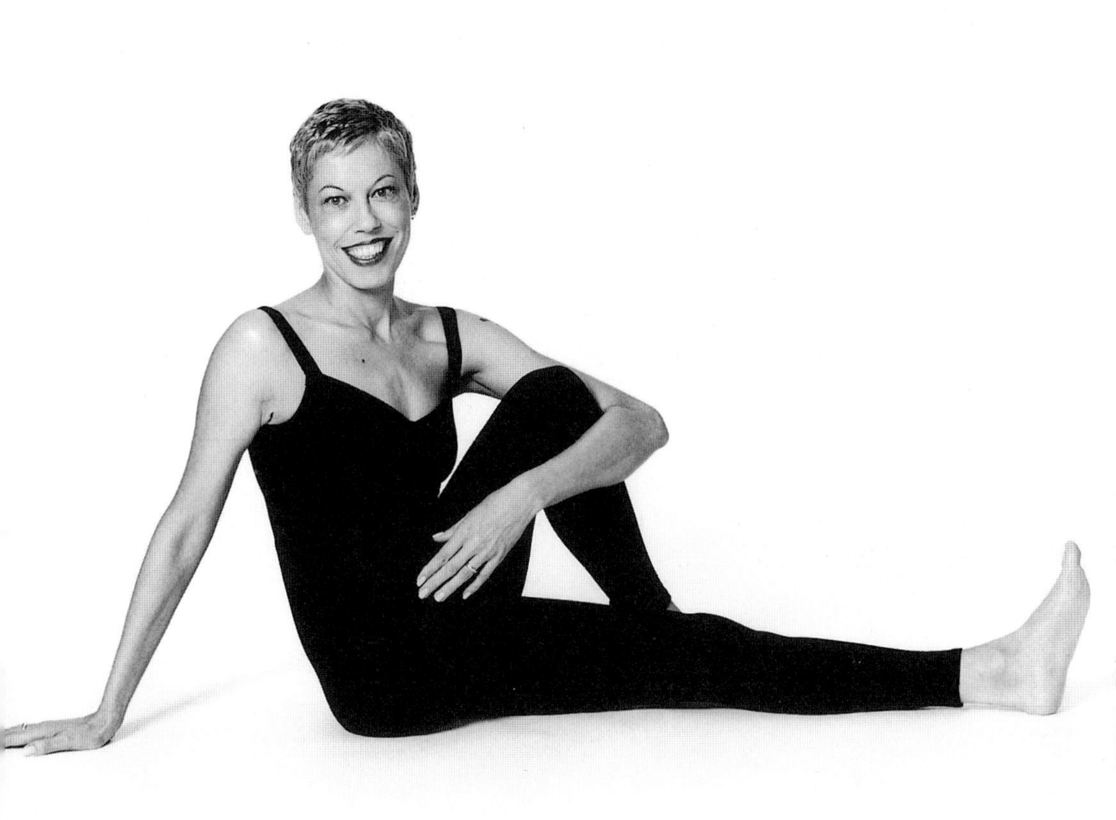

Morning maintenance for bad backs

Exercise 5.
Basic Back Exercise

Lie face down, stomach on the floor. Relax your head to the side. Gently breathe in, and feel your stomach drop to the floor. Breathe out, pull your stomach into your spine so that your tailbone drops. Don't grip your bottom or tense your shoulders. Eventually you will be able to get your fingers in between your stomach and the floor as you breathe out. Feel your stomach working.

Repeat 10 times.

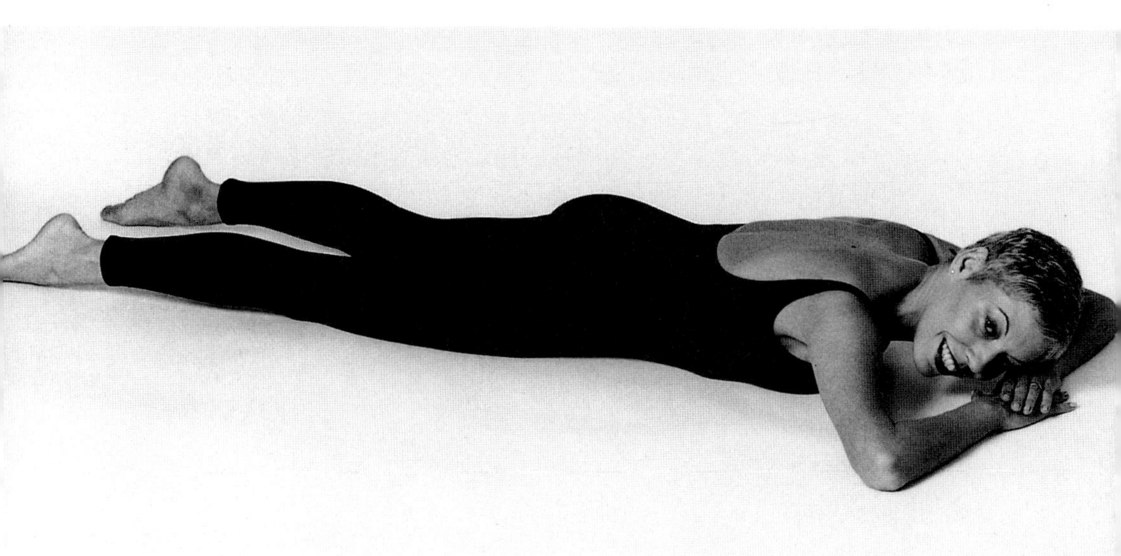

Morning maintenance for bad backs

Exercise 6.

Spine Release Exercise

Roll over onto your back. Breathe in, then very gently breathe out and, bending both knees to your chest, curl your head towards your knees. Hold, breathe in, then breathe out, and relax your head down, pulling your stomach into your spine. This is a passive back and neck stretch to stretch out your back.

Do 10 repetitions.

WATCHPOINT

Don't tense your shoulders, keep your bottom on the floor.

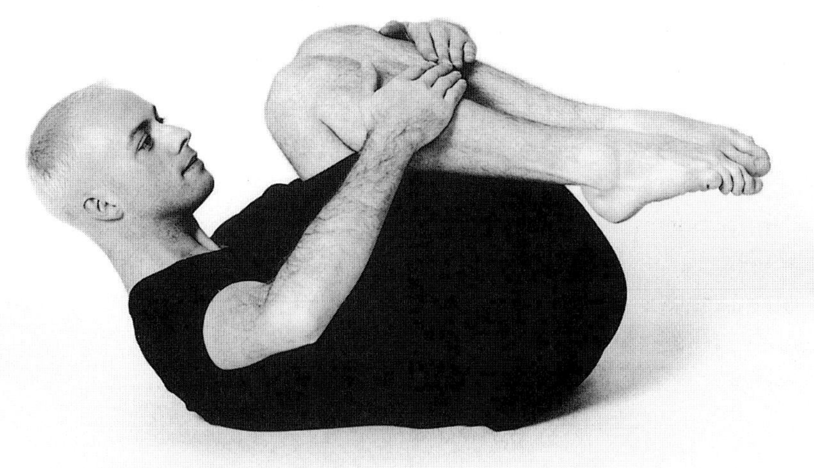

Morning maintenance for bad backs

Back surgery

Stephen Anson has been taking classes with Lesley Ackland since 1987. In 1992, he had back surgery for a herniated disc. A few years later his walking was badly affected. Every morning he does 15 minutes of Pilates exercises for his back and 10 minutes for his feet.

'The exercises mobilize me after a night of sleeping in bad positions, which leave me stiff and in some pain. Even if I haven't had a bad night's sleep I find it beneficial to keep doing the exercises – given my shape, my physiology, and the surgery I've had. I also take a Body Maintenance class once a week.'

Post Surgical Exercises

'When I went into surgery for my back, I didn't think it would be a problem at all. In fact my surgeon said that these operations are 80 per cent successful. Unluckily I was part of the 20 per cent. The surgery stopped me from limping and enabled me to sit down. My left leg stopped atrophying. So in some ways the operation was successful, but I was never able to get back into running, which was probably a contributory factor to my injury. I have not been able to carry heavy weights since the operation. Anything involving impact, like running or riding, tennis, dancing even, is completely out of the question.

'I was told at the time of surgery I would need follow-up physiotherapy and exercises for six or maybe nine months, and that I could expect to be running after a year. That never happened.

'As soon as I had the operation I could feel I had lost the spring in my step. I didn't walk with the same elasticity. Eventually it became too painful to walk. I was 50 and I was walking like someone who was 80. The operation had changed my gait, and I now have permanent damage to the left Achilles' tendon. I finally went to the London foot hospital and I now have orthotics in both my shoes and a heel cup in the left one inside the sock.'

Foot Exercises

'The foot exercises were given to me by a physiotherapist and Lesley and I discussed them. They are similar to Pilates exercises. In all this aggravation the left leg has become weaker than the right. I do calf stretches and rising up on my feet to strengthen the muscles. Walking is much more comfortable. I can now walk three or four miles without a problem.

'Apart from the occasional pain, I have to get up early to do my back and feet exercises instead of sleeping in bed. But I know, if I do 25 minutes of Pilates six or seven mornings a week, basically life is tolerable.'

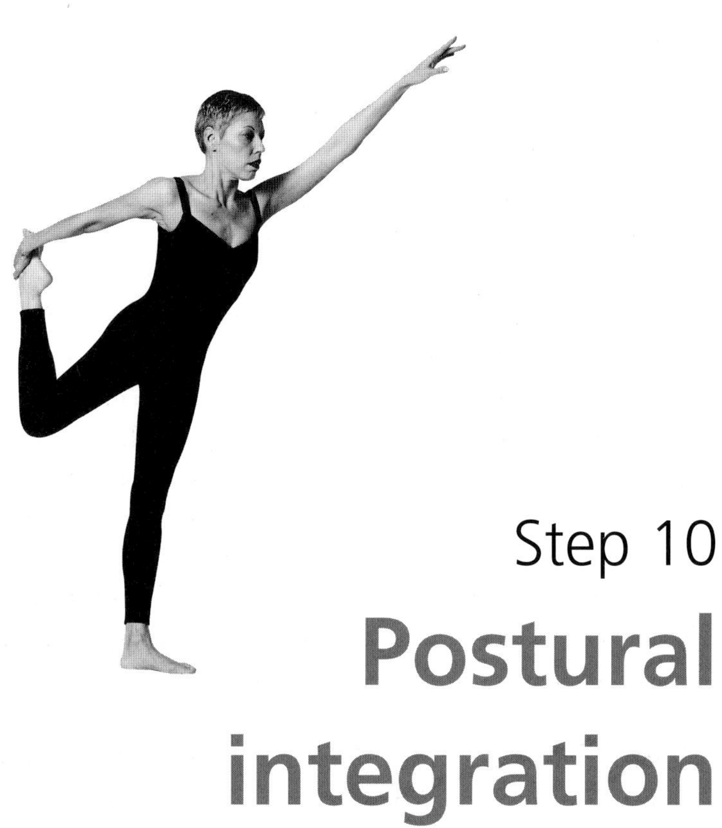

Step 10
Postural integration

This final chapter is about balance and coordination – the way we stand, the way we present ourselves. This Step will deal with standing and releasing, as well as balancing and visualization. With renewed vigour you will fight ageing and gravity, thereby presenting a positive framework – foremost to yourself, and then to others. Successfully integrating both the internal and external is difficult to accomplish, but once achieved there will be the beginning of a collaboration between the body, mind and spirit which can be tremendously empowering.

These exercises are complex, but the first exercise is reasonably straightforward and the following exercises progress from there. Obviously, while doing these exercises, you can hold on to something – a wall or a towel rail. You needn't do these exercises without some support.

The following exercises are standing balances, which get progressively harder. Start with the first one and progress slowly as your balance improves. Plan to do two exercises at a time and then take a break.

Exercise 1

Bare feet are best for this exercise. Stand with both feet grounded into the floor, the weight equally distributed over both feet, head floating, arms at your sides, tailbone dropped. Shoulders and neck are relaxed; the arms are hanging naturally in front of the body.

Don't rock forwards or backwards. Don't cling onto the floor with your toes. Very gently float one foot off the ground, hold for 10 seconds and put it down.

WATCHPOINT

When you lift that leg, make sure the pelvis is not distorted and the hips remain level.

Repeat four times, with alternating feet. Now do the same exercise with your eyes closed.

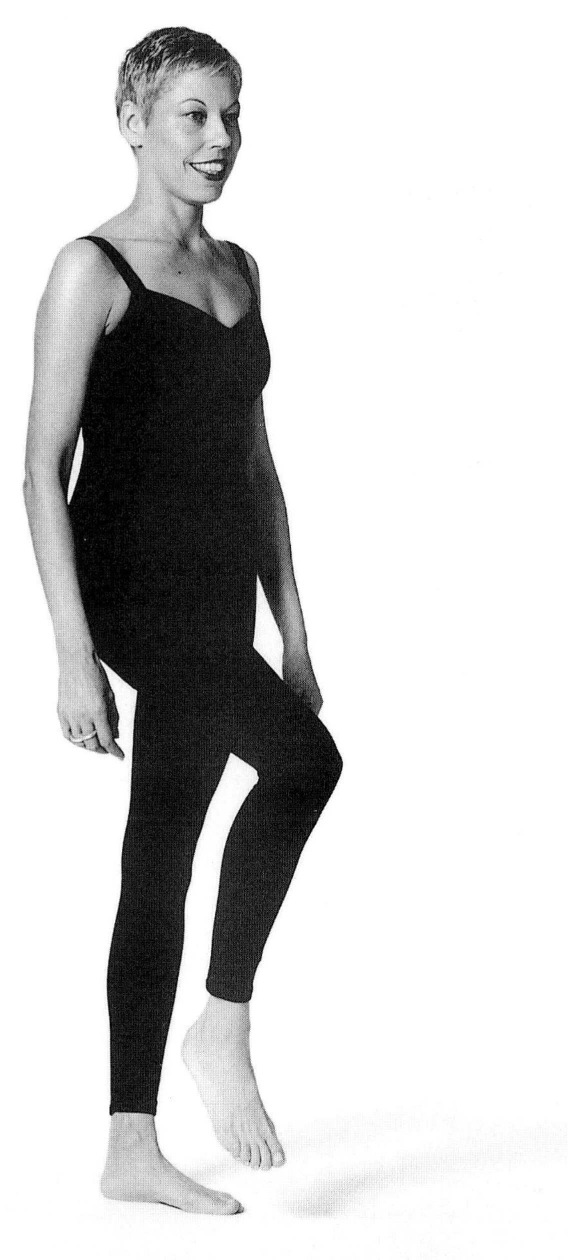

Exercise 2

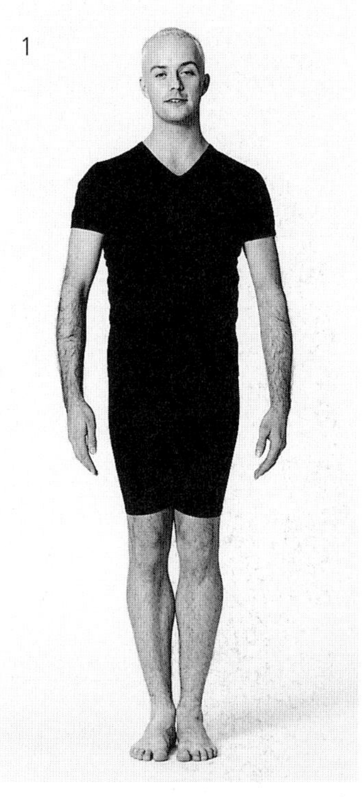

Stand with the feet close together, one foot just in front of the other.

Very gently rise onto the toes and lift one foot and place it just in front of you and come down (photograph 2).

You then rise, and lift the other foot and come down (photograph 3).

While doing this exercise it is preferable to hold on to something. If you've been doing your abdominal exercises you will feel the familiar connection of the navel to the spine. The tailbone is heavy and the head is floating, like a blossom on top of your shoulders. Your arms hang naturally beside you. Don't cling with your toes.

Take six steps forward – relax and repeat four times. When you can balance, do the exercise without holding on.

WATCHPOINT
After all the postural integration exercises, stretch your calves as explained in the Midday section.

2

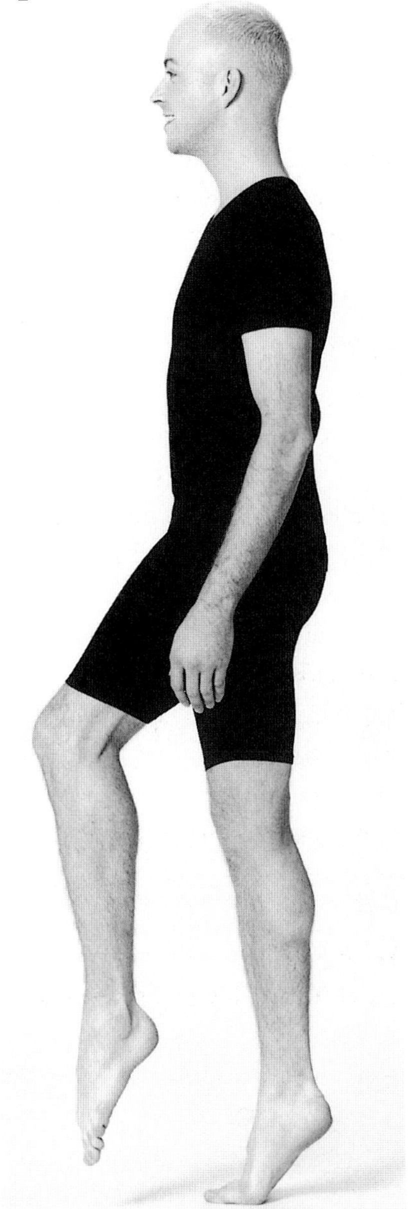

3

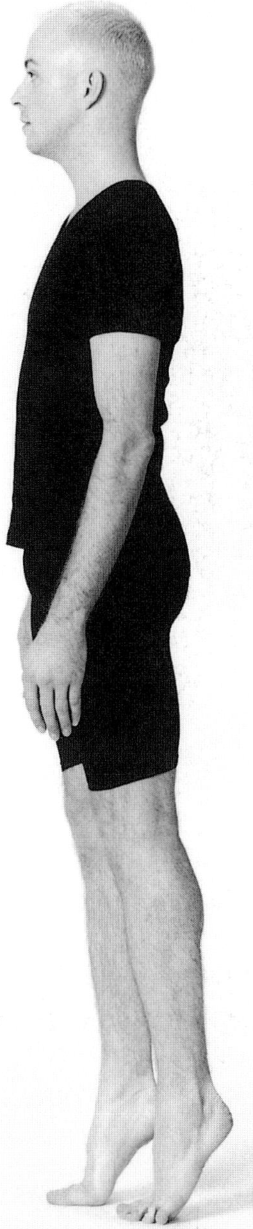

Exercise 3

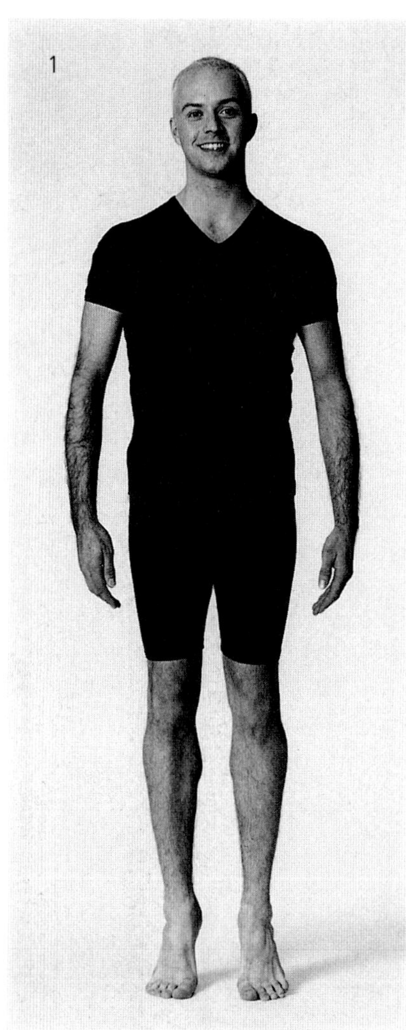

This exercise is like walking along a beam. Stand with your feet together. Rise onto the toes and take a tiny step sideways – no more than 6 inches (15 cm) distant – bring the feet together and go down. Take five little steps one way and five little steps the other.

This exercise focuses on stabilization, alignment and proprioceptive work. It will help you stand taller, move the weight out of your hips, and prevent you from sinking and slumping. You will be aware of your posture. Furthermore, this exercise will facilitate your ability to walk confidently wherever you are. Walking in crowds won't intimidate you. You will be centred, aligned and toned.

Repeat four times.

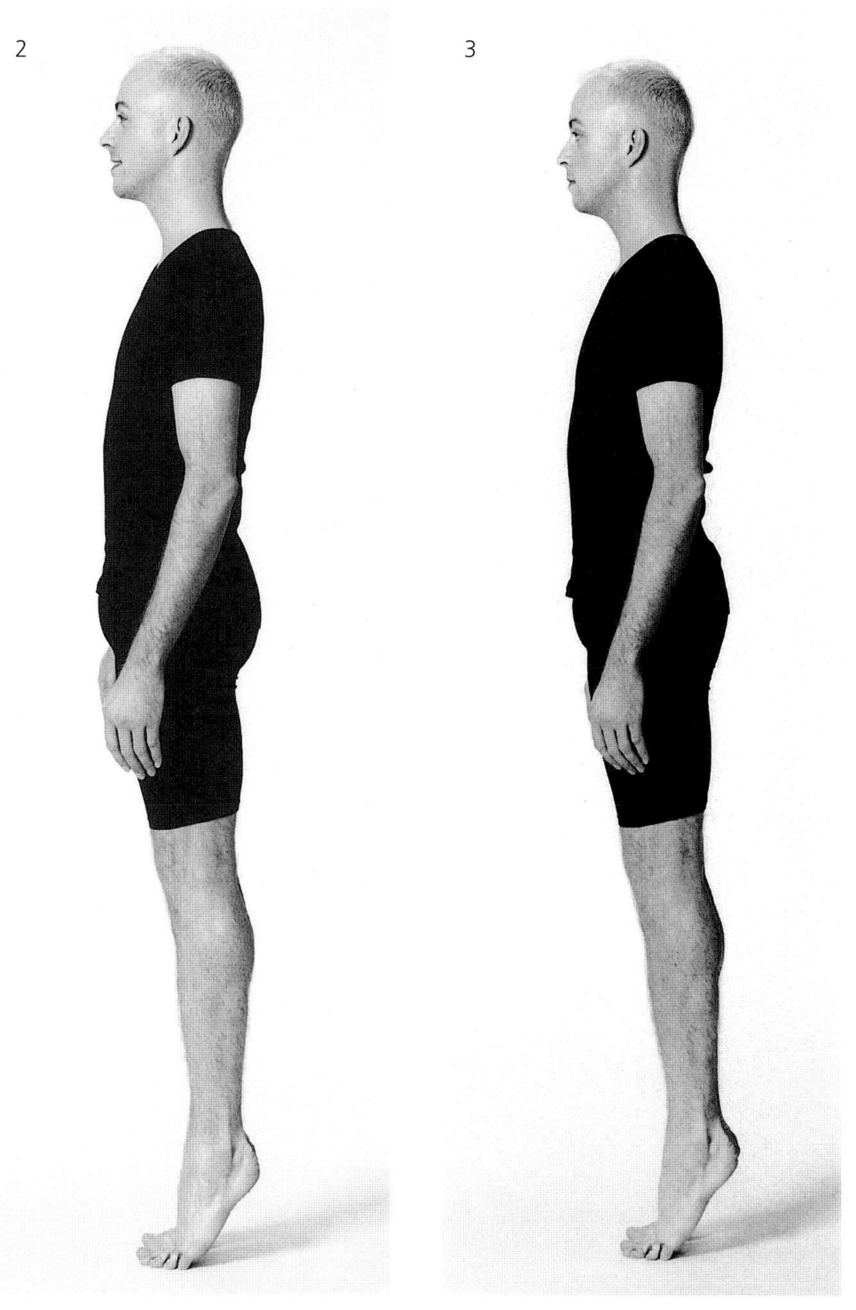
2
3

Exercise 4

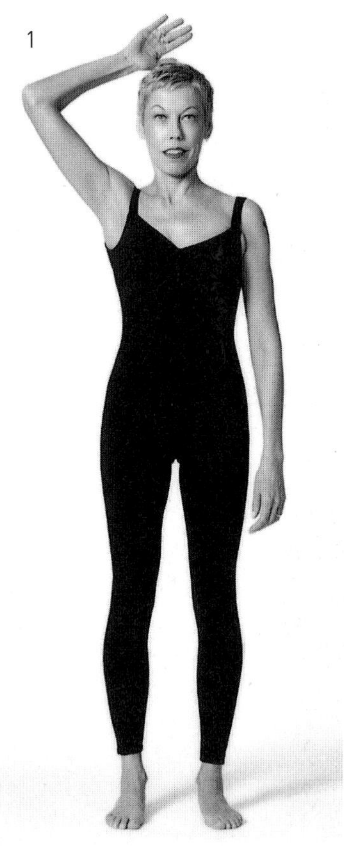

All the rules about posture apply. Your arms are beside you. Lift the right arm behind the ear and stretch it up to the crown of the head and away to the side. Breathe out as you take the movement. With your left arm, execute the same motion. The palm brushes the side of the ear and follows through to the crown of the head, up and down. It is as if you are brushing your ear away to the side of the room. Do five repetitions, alternating sides.

WATCHPOINT

Make sure the arm doesn't go behind you. You'll know if it does, as you'll feel the weight shift forward and back. Your stomach will protrude, your bottom will stick out, and your back will arch.

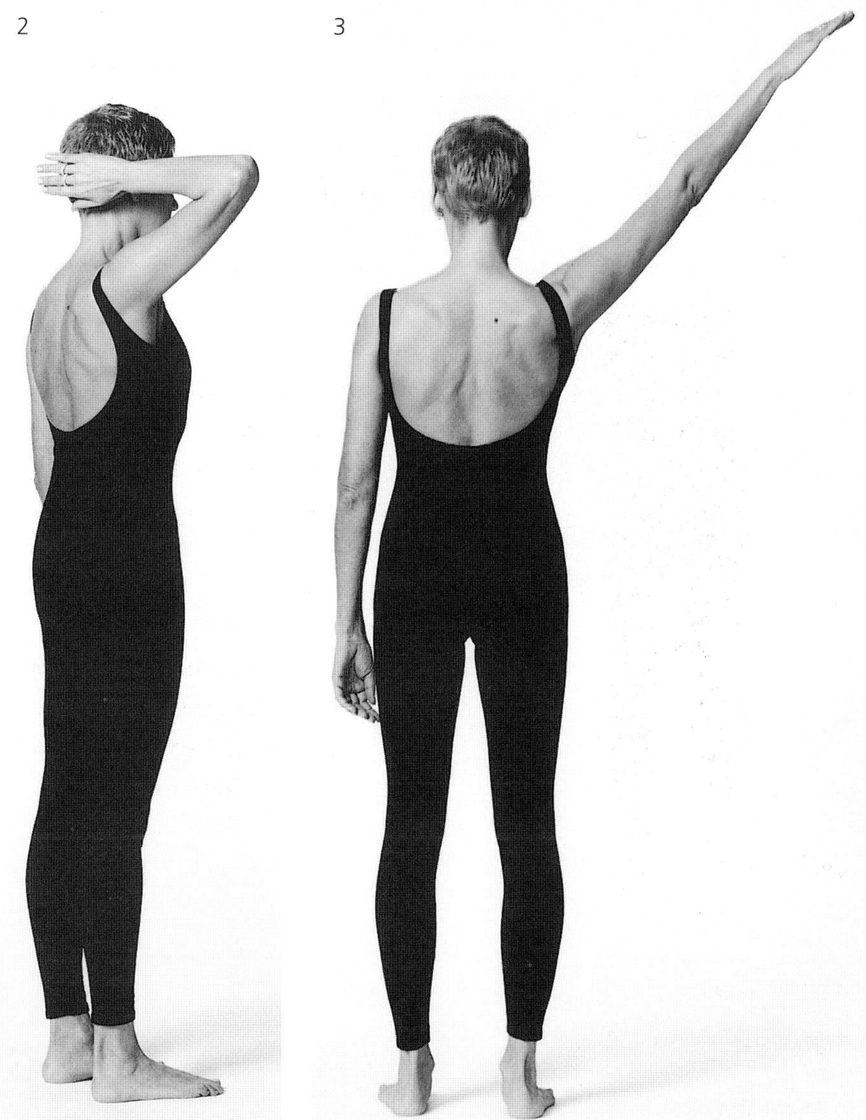
2 3

Exercise 5

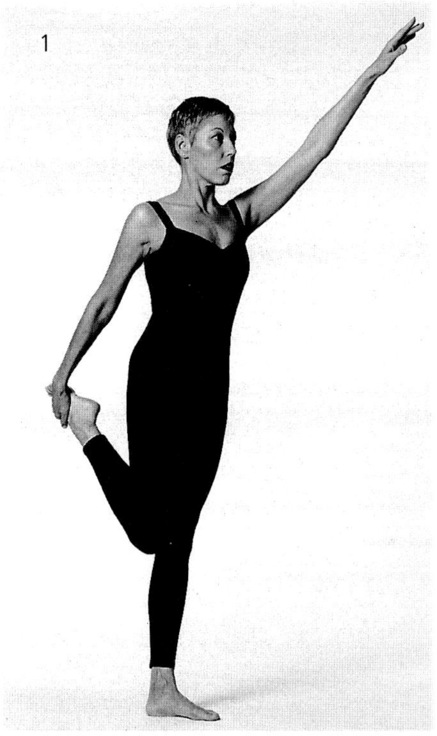

This exercise is more difficult. You should hold on to something. Stand with both feet on the ground in a starting position. Keeping the knees together, bend your right knee and with your right arm you hold on to your ankle. Bring your left arm next to your ear (photograph 1).

Stabilize that position and hold no more than 10 seconds on each leg. Do no more than four repetitions, alternating the legs. When you feel comfortable with that, you may then start to take the knee back behind you, and lean your body forward, keeping your stomach in and the tailbone dropped (photograph 2). An arched back and protruding stomach will indicate a lack of core stability needed to hold the position.

Eventually when you have that core stability you can let go of your foot and take the arms to the side during this exercise.

WATCHPOINT

There should be no pinching whatsoever in the lumbar spine during this exercise. If you do feel any pinching, it may be attributed to an incorrect pelvic alignment, tightness in your bottom or thighs, or lack of enough core strength to hold this position.

2

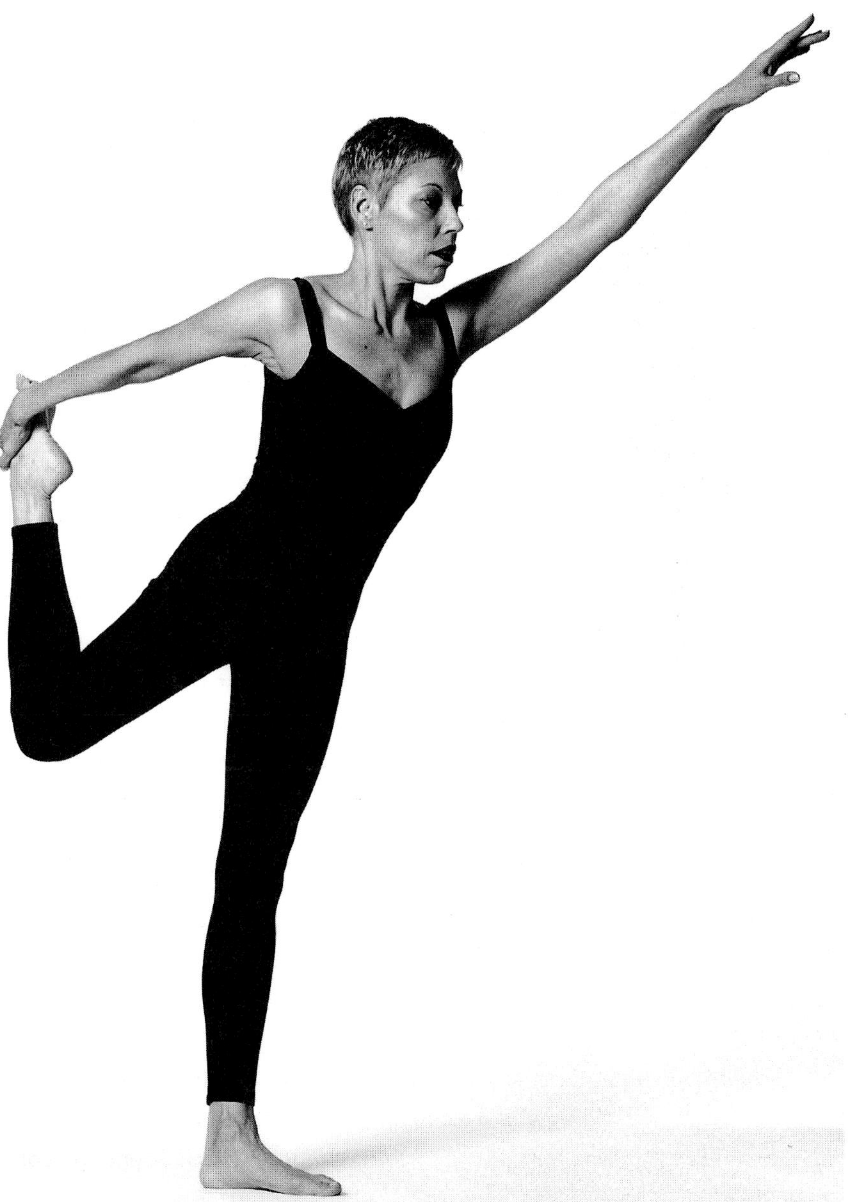

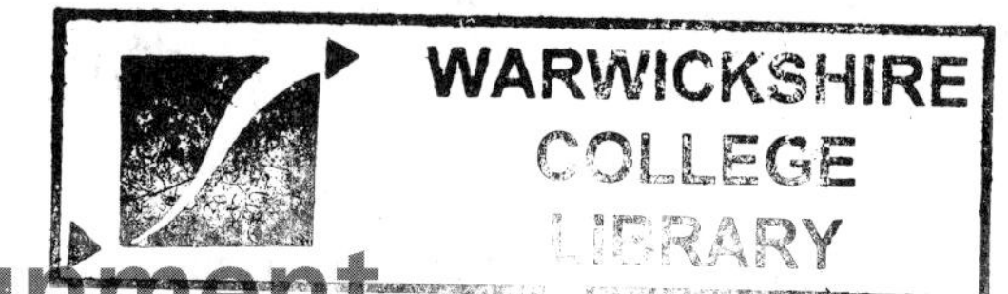

Postural realignment

Contemporary dancer and assistant artistic director of Adventures in Motion Pictures, a dance theatre company, Etta Murfitt began Pilates when she was training at the London Contemporary Dance School in 1983. She discontinued Pilates for several years, came back briefly, then stopped again. Earlier this year, she returned to Body Maintenance.

'When my baby was five-and-a-half months old, I went straight back into dancing. I assumed my body was just going to catch up with me, and it did. But I wasn't working in a particularly healthy way. I would do an intense period of dancing and rehearsal directing, and then I would do nothing except for office work and then straight back into intense dancing and rehearsing. I wouldn't do anything in between except for the odd technique class. I actually thought, "hang on a minute, I have to reassess how I work. I need something that's going to keep me ticking over and get me working in the right way."'

Deep Internal Muscles

'Pilates made me step back into myself. Instead of worrying about my external appearance I began to focus on myself internally. Pilates has centred me and has made me more aware of my deeper, internal muscles. It makes you concentrate on all those important things. When I went to Los Angeles for a performance I was able to think about all the things I needed to do in order to get through the show – i.e. pulling in my stomach, lifting and being very careful because I have Achilles Tendonitis. Doing my Pilates exercises before each show helped me enormously. I really worked with my feet to ensure that I wasn't going to worsen my injury. In fact, my feet have got much stronger.

'For all dancers, posture is extremely important, for me, even more so. Pilates has helped me with postural realignment. I've never had a particularly easy body. My shoulders are really rounded, which makes dancing difficult. A dancer must stand impossibly straight, with shoulders down at all times. People are not naturally built like that. We're built with curves in our spines.

If you look at dancers, their backs look really flat.

'The key to my postural realignment has been the work I have done with my stomach. This definitely helps because I feel lengthening through the stomach. Then everything is as it should be: your ribs fall, your shoulders drop, just through that simple pulling up through the stomach. It really transforms your posture.'

Contemporary Dance

'Contemporary dance is not vastly different from classical since most contemporary dancers train in classical technique. It is slightly better for the back – because you deal with more exercises which strengthen the back, ensuring that it is loose as well. Contemporary dance uses the back and stresses suppleness as well as strength.

'It's always experimental, so you never rely only on classical dance steps. You're always making up weird steps, which can put a lot of strain on your back and body because you are doing things that are not the norm. You could say contemporary and classical are as demanding as each other.

'Traditionally dancers have injuries. I blame not only the difficulty of the steps but the constant repetition. All the time in rehearsal, you repeat the same moves. So there's the repetitive stress of just doing class every day. The exercises serve the purpose of helping you to perform, but they constantly put wear and tear on the body, and you begin to rely on your strength. If you have a strong right leg then you tend to work that more because it feels OK, whereas if you have a funny ankle on your left leg you work that less. Pilates strengthens weakened muscles and, as a result, you have a more balanced body.'

Changing Direction

'When you're dancing you have to change direction all the time. Simultaneously you're also changing your weight. If you're strong in your centre you can do that. But if you're holding yourself incorrectly and you need to make all those quick change of directions, you can easily fall over. If I do Pilates before a dance class, just balancing on one leg is so much easier because I've already found the connection between my mind and body.'

Conclusion

Everybody's potential is limitless. Yet few of us achieve all of what we are capable. We are given boundaries, and we tend to accept them without question. There is now more equality in gender and career diversification. More importantly, we can look forward to ageing well, living longer and having more productive lives.

We often pay no attention to our bodies until something goes wrong. The human body is a splendid vehicle. In addition to our physical beings, it houses our emotional and spiritual selves. Like a car, it requires regular maintenance, especially since it can't be traded in. Our bodies remain with us all our lives. It is not costly or painful to respect and maintain them.

With *10-Step Pilates*, the Body Maintenance way, you can slowly re-create a sense of physical vitality and core stability, and look forward to continued well-being and health.